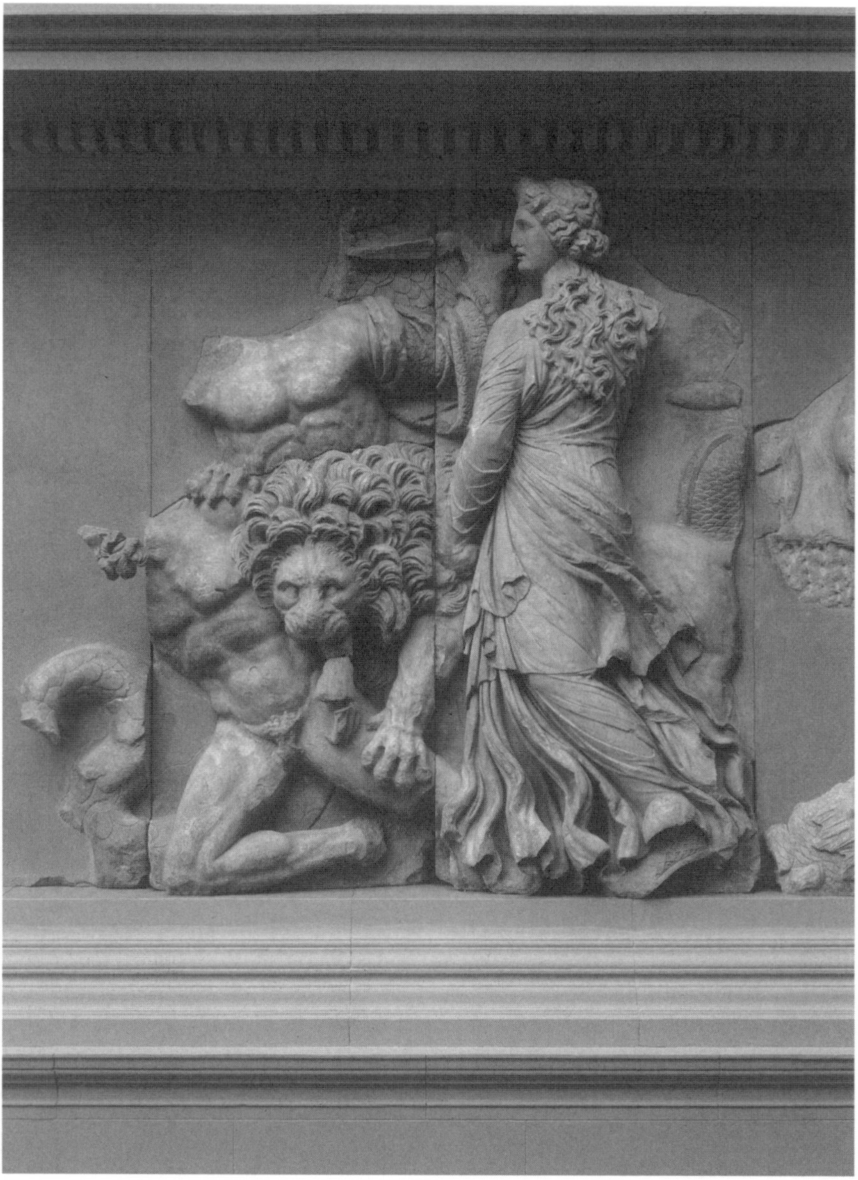

"Lion Goddess" fighting a giant. The goddess is possibly Keto, mother of the Graiae, who are walking away to the left (missing).

Hellenistic relief, 164–156 BCE
Antikensammlung, Staatliche Museen zu Berlin

Frontispiece photo credit: Bildarchiv Preussicher, Kulturbesitz/Art Resource, NY

Psychodynamics and Psychotherapy of Pseudoseizures

Dalma Kalogjera-Sackellares, PhD

Crown House Publishing
www.crownhouse.co.uk

First published by

Crown House Publishing Ltd
Crown Buildings, Bancyfelin, Carmarthen, Wales, SA33 5ND, UK
www.crownhouse.co.uk

and

Crown House Publishing Ltd
P.O.Box 2223, Williston, VT 05495-2223, USA
www.CHPUS.com

British Library of Cataloguing-in-Publication Data
A catalogue entry for this book is available from the British Library.

ISBN 1904424279

LCCN 2003115395

Printed and bound in the UK by
Cromwell Press Ltd
Trowbridge
Wiltshire

To our patients

In recognition of their willingness to meet life courageously

In spite of the difficulties to which this book is a witness

For their sake and on their behalf

Contents

Acknowledgments

I wish to express my gratitude to the following individuals:

Dr. Frank Kobler, for having faith in me always. Dr. Kobler, now Professor Emeritus, is the founder of the Doctoral Program in Clinical Psychology at the Loyola University of Chicago.

The talented professionals and teachers in the Department of Psychiatry of the Temple University Hospital in Philadelphia where I had been an intern. Philadelphia is a great center of learning and a place which for many years has kept alive psychoanalytic and psychodynamic traditions. The present book is an attempt to keep this heritage alive and to demonstrate its continued relevance. Dr. John Benson and Dr. Thomas McDonnel are remembered.

Psychodynamic theory and therapy were at the heart of the NIMH sponsored post-doctoral fellowship in gero-psychology at the Older Adult Program of the Institute of Psychiatry of the Northwestern University Medical School. Dr. David Gutmann, founder of the program, Dr. Jerome Grunes and Dr. Jacobowitz are acknowledged.

I am especially indebted to Dr. Stanley Berent, founder and, for many years, director of the Neuropsychology Program of the Department of Psychiatry at the University of Michigan Medical Center in Ann Arbor. My intense professional involvement with pseudoseizures began there, and I was given every opportunity to excel. Dr. Berent, very generous with his time and his wide professional experience, continued as a preceptor throughout my stay there. Michigan continues for me as a place of special significance and authority.

I wish to thank Dr. Douglas Anderson, chairman of the Department of Neuroscience at the University of Florida Medical Center for creating a place for me in his department. This department pursues a wide range of scientific inquiry.

I also wish to acknowledge Dr. William Luttge, director and founder of the McKnight Brain Institute at the University of Florida.

Research Service of the Malcolm Randall Veterans Administration Medical Center is acknowledged.

I wish to express special gratitude to the Health Science Center Library at the University of Florida, as well as the VA Medical Center. Mr. Dennis Hogue who directs inter-library loan service is acknowledged for his professional excellence and commitment which enabled me to gain access to important original sources.

Dr. Michael Trimble of the National Hospital for Neurology and Neurosurgery, London, UK, is acknowledged.

Dr. Timothy Betts, director of the Seizure Clinic and professor at the University of Birmingham Medical School, and an international expert in the field is acknowledged for his consistent support of my work over the years which includes, most recently, his efforts to help my life's work see the light of day. I remain most appreciative of the transatlantic accolades which are somewhat in the nature of a talisman against a rainy day.

Helen Kinsey, Acquisitions Editor at Crown House Publishing is especially acknowledged for her support and all her efforts to see my work published.

A great deal is owed to my husband and colleague Dr. J. Chris Sackellares who provided continuity in our professional and personal lives. He also provided critical feedback for this book.

The learned staff at the Pergamum Museum in Berlin as well as Cyprus Museum in Nicosia for their help in making the images of two remarkable works of Hellenistic art available to me: Head of a Young Lady and Lion Goddess Fighting a Giant.

These works were chosen for their exceptional beauty and in celebration of a tradition which considers beauty important. They exemplify what this author has termed "the therapeutic agency of beauty".

Foreword

This is a book about the psychodynamics and treatment of patients with psychogenic pseudoseizures. It is the product of years of intensive work dedicated to understanding the psychological features and the underlying psychodynamic mechanisms and to the formulation and testing of an effective therapeutic approach. To understand the psychodynamics of patients with psychogenic pseudoseizures, it was necessary to evaluate a very large number of patients with a well-established diagnosis of pseudoseizures, with a variety of diagnostic tools, and to follow a subset of these patients over extended periods of time.

A famous German writer, Georg Christian Lichtenberg, is said to have questioned why it never struck researchers that discoveries could be made not only with a magnifying glass, but also, perhaps with a diminishing lens (cited in Ferenczi, 1927). In her investigations into the problem of pseudoseizures, the author used a "magnifying glass" to examine the details in each case. However, to an even larger extent, she relied on capturing the large constellations generated by groupings of clinical features presented by the patient population as a whole ("diminishing lens" approach).

There has been a trend in pseudoseizure scholarship to search for a single mechanism which is of decisive importance. The strength of the author's approach is to demonstrate family resemblance among different presentations of the syndrome (the importance of not missing the forest for the trees).

It was necessary to evaluate a large number of patients because of the wide range of psychological complaints, signs and symptoms found in these patients. At first glance, it appears that one is dealing with a common symptom (pseudoseizures) resulting from a large number of different psychological disorders. However, through a careful study, using all of the diagnostic tools at her disposal, the author was able to identify common themes and patterns which permitted her to formulate a few well-defined syndromes, thus substantially reducing the great complexity of the clinical material.

It is also important to point out that this work is based upon evaluation of patients with a well-established diagnosis of pseudoseizures. Establishing a confident diagnosis of pseudoseizures in a large number of patients, in a reasonable period of time, is a task that could not have been achieved until some time around 1980. Up until that time, neurologists had to rely primarily upon the history provided by the patient, members of the family, or close friends. Observing a pseudoseizure first-hand was a chance occurrence which was, unfortunately, all too rare. However, with the institution of long-term EEG-video monitoring as a diagnostic tool, it became possible to record representative examples of a patient's seizures (and/or pseudoseizures). This tool provided the opportunity to analyze videotaped recordings to study the fine details of the patient's behavior during the event and to analyze the electroencephalogram (EEG) for extended periods, including the crucial period just before, during, and just after each event. This new technology taught the neurologist an important lesson in humility: even the best clinician can misdiagnose a pseudoseizure as an epileptic seizure or mistake an epileptic seizure for a psychogenic pseudoseizure. Armed with this new diagnostic tool, a number of clinical investigators began to investigate this troublesome problem, the psychogenic pseudoseizure. Now that we could identify the pseudoseizure with some degree of confidence, we could provide our psychological colleagues with a well-defined group of patients, based on an accurate diagnosis of the presenting symptom.

The author's psychological insights about pseudoseizures are derived from a very diverse range of methods (psychotherapy, neuropsychological testing, and personality testing). The diagnostic evaluations were performed personally by the author, using a diagnostic protocol established in the Neuropsychology Program at the University of Michigan. Each tool helped to describe a different aspect of this multifaceted disorder. One of the key contributions, from which she drew heavily, was extensive clinical histories obtained during interviews with the patients.

The author was thus confronted, from the beginning, with information as diverse as motor speed and grip, on the one hand, and Minnesota Multiphasic Personality Inventory profiles and psychodynamic themes emerging from the Rorschach on the other. Information emerging from extensive evaluations of this kind necessarily contains a great deal of richness. It resists strongly any attempt to reduce it rashly to a single parameter or a single issue. The author's approach was based on the decision to admit whatever was there and to understand as much of each individual component as was possible, thus letting each emerging issue speak for itself, as it were, without forcing spurious unity. This kind of approach requires that the clinician tolerate some degree of uncertainty which stems from different issues existing side-by-side, without an obvious connection. Some of the results of personality and neuropsychological testing have been published as original articles in peer-reviewed journals.

We might say that pseudoseizure syndromes are a large canvass disorder. This book helps to deal with some of the issues which make it so. A large canvass disorder requires that we accept whatever information has been obtained reliably and not exclude any, or attempt to translate one type of information into another. It is not one insight, as opposed to another, but one insight in connection with another.

In Dr. Kalogjera-Sackellares's investigations into the nature of pseudoseizures, insights and information derived from psychotherapy hold a special place. A subset of pseudoseizure patients was followed in psychotherapy over extended periods of time (months, and in some cases, years). While it is customary to think of therapy as treatment, it is really, in an equal measure, an investigation (true to its historical origins). The capacity to follow patients over time provided her with a temporal perspective that proved to be of great value in understanding this disorder. Without this longitudinal perspective, it would not have been possible to gain an appreciation for the chronicity of the disorder and the frequently changing and evolving clinical features.

This book will prove useful to psychologists, psychiatrists, neurologists, and other professionals who are engaged in the diagnosis and treatment of patients with psychogenic pseudoseizures. In the text, sophisticated psychological concepts and technical terms are explained with a clarity of language that renders it accessible to neurologists with little psychological training. For psychologists and other readers who may not be familiar with some of the diagnostic issues involved in distinguishing epileptic from pseudoseizures and the diagnostic tools used for that purpose by neurologists, I will provide a brief summary.

Psychogenic pseudoseizures are transient paroxysmal events during which the patient experiences symptoms and exhibits behaviors similar to those symptoms and behaviors that occur in epileptic seizures. Pseudoseizures can mimic many different types of epileptic seizures, most commonly complex partial or tonic-clonic seizures. Unlike epileptic seizures, pseudoseizures are not associated with organized paroxysmal rhythmic discharges in the EEG. The epileptic seizure occurs because massive numbers of neurons in the cerebral cortex and connecting structures fire off in rhythmic synchronized patterns for periods of a few seconds (in the case of an absence or myoclonic seizure) or several minutes (more typical of complex partial and tonic-clonic seizures). In contrast, there is no characteristic change in the EEG during pseudoseizures. During pseudoseizures, the EEG usually reveals a pattern of electrical activity that is typical of the alert waking state. Thus, there is no known physiological basis for these seizures. Consequently, they have been ascribed to psychological causes and, historically, classified as a conversion disorder. Contributing biological factors have been suspected, but the role and nature of these factors remains to be elucidated.

The pseudoseizure gets its name from the striking resemblance between the experiential and behavioral manifestations of the event to the experiential and behavioral manifestations of certain types of epileptic seizures. As with many poorly understood disorders, there has been much disagreement as to what to call it. In the early days of modern medicine, it was called, "hysterical seizure" or "hysteroepilepsy". In fact, the term hysterical seizure persisted as the preferred term until quite late in the 20th century. The term "psychogenic pseudoseizure" was suggested because this term did not imply an association with the condition of hysteria. However, in the 1980s an even more etiology-neutral term, "nonepileptic seizures" was popularized. Aside from being neutral with respect to etiology, the term, "nonepileptic seizure", eliminates the "pseudo", thus emphasizing the fact that it is indeed a real phenomenon and is not under the control of the patient. This latter point is important because patients with this disorder often are mistakenly diagnosed as malingerers. In this book, the author has chosen the term "psychogenic pseudoseizure" to emphasize the importance of psychological mechanisms and features.

In the context of this discussion it is helpful to point out that hysteria is a very old concept. The idea that some seemingly organic disorders lack an organic basis is one of the oldest insights in medicine. Accompanying this insight is a great deal of frustration which arises when clinicians are forced to confront the "as if" quality of hysterical disturbances, as well as their mimetic character.

A study of hysterical disturbances is one of the longest lines of clinical inquiry. These lines of inquiry have generated a wealth of information and scholarship. The study of pseudoseizures is historically contained largely within the confines of the study of hysteria. The scope of that scholarship, its controversies, as well as its contributions to our understanding of pseudoseizures, however, are not going to be pursued in the context of this book.

Pseudoseizures may resemble virtually all types of epileptic seizures, including simple partial, complex partial, partial seizures evolving to bilateral tonic-clonic (secondarily generalized) seizures, absence seizures, atypical absence seizures, tonic seizures, clonic seizures, tonic-clonic seizures, atonic seizures, and mixed forms of generalized seizures. While there are features of the pseudoseizure that differ from those of its epileptic seizure counterpart, the resemblance is so strong that most patients with pseudoseizures are diagnosed as having epileptic seizures and are sent to epileptologists and other neurologists with the diagnosis of uncontrolled epileptic seizures after having failed to respond to multiple anticonvulsant drugs.

Pseudoseizures may resemble convulsive seizures such as the primary generalized tonic-clonic seizure or the partial (focal onset) seizure with secondary generalization. In such cases, the pseudoseizure is characterized by bilateral involuntary stiffening of the trunk and extremities and/or bilateral involuntary jerking of the limbs. If standing, the patient will usually fall to the floor. Even when the patient is in a sitting or lying position at the onset, he or she is often propelled to the floor. In some instances, there are contortions of the trunk and neck, pelvic thrusting and thrashing about of the extremities. In some cases, extreme postures such as the classical arc de circle or the fetal position are assumed in the course of the event. Typically, the patient does not respond appropriately to the environment during these seizures. There may be vocalizations such as moaning, screams, shouts, or repetitive phrases. Often, the convulsive type of pseudoseizure will last a minute or so, abate, then start up again. This sequence can go on for hours, in a state resembling status epilepticus. These seizures, particularly when they occur in sequences for extended periods of time are highly dramatic and quite disconcerting to the observer. More often than not, emergency services are called in and the patient is transported to an emergency department. There, the patient is treated as if in status epilepticus. It rare instances, the patient is even intubated so as to ensure ventilation while large doses of intravenous anticonvulsant drugs are administered.

Other pseudoseizures can resemble complex partial seizures. In these cases, there may be dramatic posturing and thrashing about, and the person may remain in a sitting or standing position. Often, there is altered responsiveness to the environment, with the eyes fixed in a vacant stare, or looking aimlessly about, giving the appearance of confusion or bewilderment. The patient may appear frightened, and may cry out, shout, or scream. There may be no responses to questions or statements by the observer, or the responses may appear inappropriate. The patient may moan, sob, or repeat words or phrases. There may be involuntary repetitive automatic behaviors such as rocking back and forth or fiddling with clothing, utensils, or other objects. The episodes can last seconds to hours. Like convulsive seizures, the complex partial-like pseudoseizures can occur in series, giving an appearance of complex partial status. Like complex partial seizures, the patient generally has no recall of the event.

The diagnostic difficulty is further complicated by the fact that a substantial portion of patients with psychogenic pseudoseizures also have epilepsy. In fact, it has been reported by some epilepsy centers that as many as 25% of patients with pseudoseizures have concomitant epilepsy (Kalogjera-Sackellares and Sackellares 1997a, 1997b). Thus, patients with psychogenic pseudoseizures are about 20 times more likely to have epilepsy than the general population. Consequently, documenting a pseudoseizure with EEG-video monitoring does not exclude the diagnosis of epilepsy; it makes it more likely. This point becomes quite relevant when formulating plans for clinical management.

In the typical case, a patient with pseudoseizures will be initially diagnosed with epilepsy. Based on this diagnosis, he or she is treated with a series of anticonvulsant drugs, both as single agents and in combination. When the treatment fails, doses are increased to higher and higher levels. After persistent therapeutic failure, the patient may be referred to other physicians. Actually, it is often the patient who initiates a change in physicians and consults with other physicians. Ultimately, the patient is evaluated by multiple physicians and subjected to multiple EEG recording sessions and neuroimaging procedures. Finally, the patient is referred to an epilepsy center for medically intractable epilepsy.

In many instances, by the time the patient reaches the epilepsy center, he or she has been symptomatic for several years (even decades) and the disorder has caused major disruption in quality of life for the patient, family and friends, and the community. In addition, there is usually a string of frustrated physicians along the way. In many cases, the diagnosis of pseudoseizures is not determined until the patient has been admitted to hospital for presurgical evaluation.

The presurgical evaluation is aimed toward classifying the seizure type, determining if the seizures originate locally in one cerebral hemisphere, and to localize the seizure onset zone. The initial evaluation, called Phase I of the evaluation, includes special magnetic resonance imaging (MRI) scans, positron emission tomography (PET) scans, one or more long-term EEG-video recordings of the patient (a lengthy inpatient procedure lasting days to as much as 3 weeks), and an extensive neuropsychological test battery. Neuroimaging procedures are performed to find evidence of a structural lesion in the brain. Many types of medically refractory seizures are due to localized structural lesions that are epileptogenic. Such lesions include mesial temporal sclerosis, developmental malformations, lesions caused by traumatic brain injury, stroke, or resolved meningitis or encephalitis. Most of these lesions can be demonstrated with modern MRI procedures.

EEG-video monitoring procedures are performed to look for interictal (between seizures) epileptiform discharges and to record the clinical and EEG manifestations of several typical seizures. The objective of the neuropsychological test battery is to identify motor and cognitive deficits in order to localize areas of the cerebral cortex that are not functioning normally. In many centers, personality inventories and psychometric instruments aimed at detecting evidence of depression, anxiety, personality disorders, and psychoses are administered as part of the evaluation.

When Phase I presurgical monitoring is completed the results are reviewed and discussed by an interdisciplinary diagnostic and treatment team. This team usually consists of neurologists with special expertise in epilepsy and clinical neurophysiology, neuroradiologists, neurosurgeons with special expertise in epilepsy and stereotactic surgery, and neuropsychologists. The team uses information obtained through clinical interviews of the patient and family members, findings on neuroimaging tests, results of the neuropsychological testing, and results from the EEG-video monitoring procedures to establish a diagnosis and come to a conclusion. Of these procedures, the EEG-video monitoring results are most crucial in establishing the diagnosis of epilepsy or psychogenic pseudoseizures.

The Phase I EEG-video monitoring procedure involves continuous recording of the EEG from scalp and sphenoidal electrodes over a period of days to weeks. The primary objective of the procedure is to record a sample of the patient's typical seizures. To accomplish this, doses of anticonvulsant medications are reduced. In some instances the medications are discontinued. In some instances, patients may experience two or more different clinical seizure patterns.

Several lines of evidence are employed to make the diagnosis. First, the interictal (between seizure) EEG is sampled extensively to look for interictal patterns (e.g. spikes or spike and wave complexes occurring in temporal or frontal electrodes) that occur in patients with epilepsy. These interictal epileptiform patterns are common in patients with epilepsy, but occur only rarely in individuals who do not have epilepsy. Since psychogenic pseudoseizures can occur in patients with epilepsy, documenting interictal epileptiform discharges does not rule out the possibility that the patient has psychogenic pseudoseizures. Conversely, the absence of interictal epileptiform activity does not rule out epilepsy and cannot be used to establish the diagnosis of psychogenic pseudoseizures.

The strongest diagnostic evidence for epileptic seizures or psychogenic pseudoseizures comes from analysis of segments of the EEG-video recording that begin a few minutes before each seizure onset and continue until several minutes after the seizures. This perictal period is analyzed in detail. The patient's behavior patterns before, during, and after the seizure are analyzed to determine whether the clinical manifestations of the event are consistent with epileptic seizures. This information also is used to classify the seizure type. There are some features that are more typical of epileptic seizures than of psychogenic pseudoseizures, and vice versa. For example, there are rare features, such as forceful voluntary eye closure, and certain patterns of involuntary motor behavior (e.g. simultaneous jerking of left arm and right leg, but not right arm and left leg), that never, or almost never, occur during epileptic seizures, but commonly occur in psychogenic pseudoseizures. In contrast, urinary or fecal incontinence and tongue-biting rarely occur during pseudoseizures.

The perictal EEG is also analyzed visually, in great detail. Epileptic seizures are due to a paroxysmal organized discharge of cortical neurons. This discharge usually involves a sufficient area of cerebral cortex to generate electrical potentials that can be recorded from electrodes placed on the scalp. Thus, most epileptic seizures are accompanied by characteristic ictal EEG patterns. Also, there are characteristic EEG changes that are present immediately after the seizure, referred to as postictal patterns. The postictal EEG usually shows a marked drop in the EEG voltage, absence of faster rhythms and preponderance of slow wave activity. In psychogenic pseudoseizures, the EEG does not contain ictal epileptogenic patterns nor is the postictal slowing and voltage suppression observed after a psychogenic pseudoseizure.

In most instances, the combined information obtained from the interictal and perictal EEG, ictal video analysis of the patient during the seizure, supported by information obtained through clinical interviews, neuroimaging procedures, and neuropsychological testing is sufficient to diagnose and classify epileptic seizures and to detect the occurrences of psychogenic pseudoseizures. There are some instances when a given event cannot be classified as epileptic or psychogenic. This is particularly true in some frontal lobe seizures because the clinical behavior patterns are quite different from other types of epileptic seizures and the ictal EEG discharge cannot be recorded with scalp electrodes.

Even after seizures have been recorded in Phase I monitoring, there can be causes for diagnostic uncertainty. First, patients with pseudoseizures also can have epileptic seizures. Thus, recording an epileptic seizure does not exclude the possibility that the patient also experiences psychogenic pseudoseizures. The reverse also is true. Recording a psychogenic pseudoseizure does not exclude the diagnosis of concomitant epilepsy in that patient. To some degree, there must remain some uncertainty in the diagnosis.

The diligent and exhaustive diagnostic workup outlined in the preceding paragraphs only occurs at large epilepsy centers. However, even there, increasing restrictions imposed by third-party payers and progressively limited resources may preclude such extensive evaluations. Thus, the clinician and the patient are forced to live with even more diagnostic uncertainty.

This inherent diagnostic uncertainty is a very important issue with respect to formulating the psychological as well as the neurological treatment of patients suffering from pseudoseizures. It is quite common for the patient to receive markedly conflicting opinions from a number of physicians. Is it neurological or is it psychological? The question often is posed as a "differential diagnosis", assuming that the patient's seizures are due to one etiology or the other. If it is uncertain, the caregiver feels immobilized and frustrated. At this juncture, an alternative approach will break the impasse.

The two diagnoses—epileptic seizure versus psychogenic pseudoseizure—should not be considered as two incompatible alternatives. Rather, the neurologist must decide if there is sufficient evidence of epilepsy to institute or continue chronic anticonvulsant drug therapy, and the psychologist or psychiatrist must independently decide whether there is sufficient evidence to initiate psychiatric treatment. Often, the answer to both questions is affirmative (i.e. psychogenic pseudoseizures are confirmed, but concomitant epilepsy cannot be excluded with confidence). In these cases, anticonvulsants should be used in doses usually appropriate for seizure control, antidepressant or antianxiety drugs should be used, as indicated, if these symptoms are present, and psychotherapy should be offered to the patient.

When patients present with debilitating physical and neurological symptoms that cannot be readily explained and unrevealing diagnostic test results (e.g. EEG and MRI), it is natural to blame the patient. There is a temptation to believe, at least at some level, that the patient has the ability to control their pseudoseizures, given sufficient moral fiber and effort. This is one of the classes of disorders for which the patient is held responsible for its cause and the failure to respond to treatment. At this point, the diagnosis of malingering is often entertained. While malingering occurs, it is rare among those who present with intractable psychogenic pseudoseizures.

It is important to emphasize that the role of the neurologist is not exhausted, even after epilepsy is "ruled out" and the diagnosis of pseudoseizures is established. In truth, the uncertainty of the diagnosis requires that the neurologist remain available for periodic re-evaluation. In some instances, the diagnosis of concurrent epileptic seizures is established months to years after the diagnosis of psychogenic pseudoseizures has been made. Optimal care of these patients involves close collaboration between neurology, clinical psychology, and psychiatry.

Somewhat surprisingly, establishing the diagnosis of psychogenic pseudoseizures is only the beginning of the diagnostic effort. The real challenge is to determine the nature of the underlying psychological disorder. This book is dedicated specifically to meeting this goal.

As a neurologist, my interest in and professional engagement with patients with psychogenic pseudoseizures stems from the fact that such patients represent a substantial proportion of patients referred for the diagnosis and treatment of their seizure disorder. While these patients often experience other somatic as well as psychiatric symptoms, it is the seizures that evoke the most concern. Further, it is the neurophysiologic and neuroimaging tools of the neurologist that are essential for establishing the diagnosis with any degree of certainty.

While the neurological approach is quite effective in establishing the diagnosis, it is not, at least at this juncture, useful in defining the pathophysiology or in formulating an effective treatment. Although clinical and neuropsychological investigations suggest that neurological disturbances may play a role in the pathophysiology, this idea remains a hypothesis to be tested. One cannot base treatment on working hypotheses about the psychobiology. At the present time, we cannot even formulate pharmacological interventions on the basis of empirical studies because such studies have not been done. Thus, a well-conceived approach to evidence-based pharmacotherapy has yet to be formulated.

In contrast, the psychological and psychosocial features prevalent in patients with psychogenic pseudoseizures are quite prominent. Further, there are similarities among cases that allow us to recognize the disorder and to define subtypes. These common psychological features also provide insight into the mechanisms that underlie the disorder. In this book, the author describes the common clinical patterns that define several specific syndromes found in patients presenting with psychogenic pseudoseizures. This classification scheme emphasizes the most prominent and distinguishing features of each syndrome and provides a framework for understanding the underlying psychodynamics.

The book is based upon 15 years of the author's professional engagement with this disorder. This work consisted of intensive clinical practice and clinical investigations. The work entailed comprehensive clinical and neuropsychological evaluations in scores of patients, a number of whom she treated over a span of years. This experience provided the opportunity to observe a wide range of clinical presentations as well as an opportunity to observe the clinical course as the symptoms evolved over time. This large cross-section of patients and longitudinal perspective is particularly important to the understanding of psychogenic pseudoseizures. This stems from the fact that patients present with a wide range of symptom patterns which, even in the same patient, vary over time.

As an initial step, Dr. Kalogjera-Sackellares formulated and described a classification of the clinical syndromes observed in patients presenting with psychogenic pseudoseizures. This classification scheme provides a framework for recognizing the disorder and understanding the psychodynamics. First published as a chapter in *Psychological Disturbances in Epilepsy*, (Sackellares and Berent, eds, 1996) this work is reproduced here in Section I to introduce the reader to the major clinical syndromes and to provide an overview of the key psychodynamic features important in the diagnosis and treatment of the disorder. The central feature of each syndrome is the presence of trauma. In some instances, the trauma is a single catastrophic event. In others, it is the result of chronic recurrent traumata. Thus, the key to recognizing, understanding, and treating patients with pseudoseizures is recognition of the key role of trauma and the response to trauma in the psychopathology of these patients.

In an effort to explain how trauma leads to the development of pseudoseizure syndromes, the author draws upon three major areas of psychodynamic theory: (1) psychoanalytic theory, (2) object-relations theory, and (3) self-psychology. Fundamental concepts from each of these areas are used to explain clinical symptomatology and to formulate effective therapeutic approaches.

Finally, the author presents a working model of psychogenic pseudoseizure syndromes. This model centers around three cardinal features: (1) the importance of trauma, (2) the chronicity of symptoms, and (3) the wide range of symptoms experienced by individual patients. This model provides the framework for diagnosing psychogenic pseudoseizure syndromes, conceptualizing the psychodynamics leading to the disorder, and formulating effective approaches to therapy.

The book describes a number of situations and problems commonly encountered among patients presenting with psychogenic pseudoseizures. The descriptions of these clinical scenarios will prove useful, enabling the clinician and therapist to more readily recognize them in his or her own practice. Just as helpful are the insightful "Points of Technique" that will prove invaluable to the psychotherapist. Effective interventions are described for many difficult situations commonly encountered in the course of psychotherapy.

Pseudoseizures are an understandable and treatable neuropsychiatric disorder. The author's intent is to foster interest and inquiry into the mechanisms whereby pseudoseizures are generated, and even more importantly, mechanisms that promote healing and restoration.

While this is a challenging disorder, about which much remains to be learned, it is also the case that a great deal is already known. We have at our disposal a variety of tools, among them neuropsychological and personality testing, especially Rorschach, as well as psychodynamic theory and therapy. Psychotherapy remains a powerful investigative tool in its own right. Psychodynamic theory has undergone more than 100 years of intensive development and has generated a wealth of conceptual contributions and techniques. This is a very substantial heritage.

J. Chris Sackellares, M.D.

Professor of Neurology, Psychiatry, Neuroscience,
and Biomedical Engineering
University of Florida

Staff Neurologist, Malcolm Randall Veterans
Administration Medical Center
Gainesville, Florida

Section I

Psychological Disturbances in Patients with Pseudoseizures

Reprinted from Psychological Disturbances in Epilepsy, *Sackellares, J. C. and Berent, S. (eds), Chapter Ten, Psychological Disturbances in Patients with Pseudoseizures, pp. 191–217, 1996, with permission from Elsevier.*

Introduction

It is generally known that pseudoseizures can occur as a result of psychological disturbance. Over 100 years ago, Charcot recognized such cases, and attributed them to hysterical conversion (Charcot, 1879). Through the years, it has become clear that pseudoseizures can occur in the context of a number of psychological disorders. Based on my own work at the University of Michigan Medical Center, I have found that there are two major etiologic categories that account for the majority of pseudoseizure cases: Post-Traumatic Pseudoseizure Syndrome and Developmental Pseudoseizure Syndrome (Table 1 below). It is important to recognize these two syndromes because they represent different psychological difficulties. Understanding these difficulties and the psychodynamic processes that underlie them is essential for formulating an effective therapeutic approach.

Classification of pseudoseizure syndromes

Table 1: Classification of pseudoseizure syndromes

1. Post-traumatic pseudoseizure syndrome
   a. Sexual trauma
   b. Trauma due to head injury or post-concussive state
   c. Chronic traumatic life course

2. Developmental pseudoseizure syndrome

Post-traumatic pseudoseizure syndrome

In this general category, pseudoseizures develop in response to a traumatic experience (or many) that the patient cannot adequately process or integrate given his or her overall psychological resources. The trauma can be recent (for example, a motor vehicle accident) or distant in time (sexual abuse in childhood). Before proceeding with the discussion of specific forms of Post-Traumatic Pseudoseizure Syndrome (PTPS) it may be useful to review the general features of the Post-Traumatic Stress Disorder (PTSD) of which PTPS is a special variant.

PTSD is found in a variety of populations. Historically, it has evolved out of studies of "traumatic neuroses of war" (Kardiner, 1959) and is, thus, intimately linked to the experiences of war veterans. More recently, this has included a study of Vietnam veterans (Schlenger et al., 1992). Finally, PTSD has been described, in its most severe and malignant form, in the victims of the Holocaust (Krystal, 1981). Krystal has studied a large number of concentration camp survivors over a long period of time and has treated some with individual analytic psychotherapy. He has amassed and integrated a large body of clinical data. In his eloquent discussion of the problems of survivors, he has described several issues that are of particular relevance to our own investigation of the PTPS (Krystal, 1981).

Krystal recognized that survivors tend to have a wide range of disturbances: affective, cognitive, and characterologic (Krystal, 1981). Thus he recognized the comprehensive nature of post-traumatic symptomatology. He described cognitive problems, persisting affective difficulties, including regression in the experience and expression of affect, anhedonia, alexithymia, a high incidence of psychosomatic disease, and general constriction of the personality. He concluded that such severe reactions tended to occur in response to "unavoidable danger", and emphasized that it was the inevitability of danger, rather than the "intensity of stimuli" that was crucial in generating post-traumatic states

(Krystal, 1981, Krystal, 1970). He linked various manifestations of PTSD, especially anhedonia and alexithymia, to the process of regression of affect, which occurs in situations of profound threat.

Krystal reviewed the well-known trajectory of affect development along three crucial dimensions: intensity, degree of differentiation, and autonomy from somatic sensation (Krystal, 1981). Briefly, early affective states are highly intense, they are global and undifferentiated (extremes of pleasure and pain), and impossible to separate from physical sensations. In the course of development, affects become expressed in gradations of intensity, they evolve into a variety of different feelings, and finally, they are experienced as separate from physical states of illness or well-being.

According to Krystal, victims of severe trauma undergo regression from the more developed to the more rudimentary forms of affective expression, which can include marked anhedonia and alexithymia. Affective states become highly restricted. Restriction of the affective range occurs because affect itself, namely, any affective experience, becomes too threatening because it cannot be separated from the memory of trauma. Clinically, this means that the patient dare not feel or remember for fear of being flooded (Krystal, 1981).

Obviously, not all features that Krystal described are manifested in pseudoseizure patients with post-traumatic states, nor do those that are present occur necessarily with the same intensity. However, he has provided a paradigm that is highly useful. He has also characterized not just the symptoms, but also the mechanisms whereby trauma generates symptoms. All of this is very pertinent to the study of pseudoseizure patients, and it provides us with a *meaning analog* or crucial parallels that we can use to organize our clinical observations.

Sexual trauma

This is a rather common feature in the histories of patients with pseudoseizures, especially among the survivors of incest (Jehu, 1991; Gross, 1982; Betts and Boden, 1992; Cartmill and Betts, 1992). Patients in this category are usually female. Sexual abuse in childhood is traumatic, both physically and psychologically, and it creates numerous difficulties which affect the way the patient thinks of herself, her attitude toward her body, and her relationships with others. A wide range of difficulties in victims of sexual abuse have been summarized by Shapiro (1991), and Browne and Finkelhor (1986). Difficulties I have found clinically to be especially common in pseudoseizure patients who are victims of sexual trauma are chronic dysphoria or lingering depressiveness, chronic anxiety, nightmares, inhibition of sexual expression or sexual anhedonia, ambivalence about affection (conflict between strong affectional needs and intense fear of closeness), withdrawal from pleasurable and productive activities, social withdrawal, and intrusive images of trauma, which can have the character of flashbacks. Dissociation is also found.

Among this wide variety of phenomena, difficulties with closeness, a sense of damage with regard to one's own body, and nightmares are very common. Fear of closeness can take the form of active avoidance of intimacy; but even more frequently, it manifests itself indirectly through anxiety, which arises in intimate situations and which can become very acute, leading to confusion or episodes of pseudoseizures. At other times, the fear of closeness can surface (again indirectly) as anger or vivid irritability, which the patient cannot link to any obvious cause. This anger is often tied to a fear of merging with others, or a fear of being retraumatized by them. Intimacy can, thus, arouse multiple anxieties, even in patients who are capable of sustained affection and loyalty toward their spouses. One can thus encounter a marked fear of intimacy alongside a very dependent personality style.

Traumatized individuals can also express fear of intimacy by acting out, or by persistently choosing partners who are not nurturant or satisfactory. Transient relationships with disappointing partners, while causing frustration, nonetheless can serve to protect the patient from deeper anxieties that intimacy can evoke (which is a well-recognized clinical pattern). In a sense, the enduring interpersonal challenge of the traumatized patient is to answer for herself the question: Is it possible to love without being victimized?

An inner sense of damage and changes in the perception of one's body are also quite common, although they are difficult to verbalize directly. More often, these feelings are expressed metaphorically: "I feel like I am in a costume all the time," or "I feel like I have 300 layers of something on me." A changed experience of one's own body is rarely brought up by the patient as a complaint. Rather, its full significance, and its prevalence, are best appreciated by analyzing the patient's spontaneous imagery and the patient's dreams. Dreams of traumatized pseudoseizure patients are distinctive in their abundant imagery of dramatic danger and damage, ranging from loss of limb, to being beheaded, being eaten by dogs or run over by a car, seeing one's house on fire, or being tormented.

Dissociation in various degrees is also found in the PTPS syndrome. Its post-traumatic origin has been recognized by a variety of authors, including Jehu (1991). An extensive discussion of the connection between sexual abuse and dissociation is provided by Davies and Frawley (1991). They have integrated an impressive amount of clinical information, and have delineated mechanisms whereby sexual abuse (especially incest) leads to severe forms of dissociation, such as dissociative personality disorder. They described, very eloquently, the arduous struggles of abuse victims with the internalized "victim-abuser" relationship paradigms, and the victims' tendency to repeat that paradigm in other significant relationships. The authors describe the defensive role dissociation plays in protecting the patient from threats of disintegration due to the impact of trauma. Davies and Frawley (1991) do not deal with pseudoseizures as such. However, their observations and conclusions are very useful and applicable in those patients whose pseudo-seizures are linked to very severe post-traumatic states, specifically patients in whom there has been a marked personality regression and subsequent reorganization of personality into a dissociative personality disorder.

The wide variety of symptomatology that has been shown to stem from the trauma can be puzzling. Mardi Horowitz, who has researched post-traumatic conditions extensively and has contributed impressively to our understanding of this area, organized the symptoms into two categories or phases: (1) the intrusive stage and (2) the phase of emotional constriction and numbing (Horowitz, 1986). The first stage is characterized by "unbidden ideas, sudden rushes of feeling and even compulsive actions, hypervigilance, startle reaction, sleep and dream disturbances, ruminations, intrusive-repetitive thoughts, feelings of being pressured, confused or disorganized when thinking about themes related to the event" (Horowitz, 1986). The second phase, which he also calls "psychic numbing", can include such features as "amnesia, daze, selective inattention, constriction of range of thought, emotional numbness and behavioral constriction" (Horowitz, 1986). In my experience, the patients with pseudoseizures tend to experience symptoms of both types in an intercurrent way, so that they may be simultaneously understimulated and overstimulated. They are understimulated in terms of lowered interest in the outside world and lower involvement in their own productive and meaningful activities, and overstimulated from within by painful memories, flashbacks, and anxiety.

As is evident from the preceding discussion, post-traumatic pseudo-seizures may present with a wide variety of symptoms that may bear no apparent relationship to the trauma which caused them (Cartmill and Betts, 1992) or to one another. This is not surprising since symptoms themselves can be so diverse, even within an individual case. Betts, who has worked extensively with pseudoseizure patients, has made an observation that the patient may not remember the trauma at all, or even if she does, may not remember its full significance, nor the relationship between the symptoms and the trauma (Cartmill and Betts, 1992). Furthermore, the victim may remember the trauma, but not the associated affect (Jehu, 1991). Consequently, one may encounter, upon initial evaluation of trauma victims, a very matter-of-fact, even flat presentation. This makes it difficult to decide whether, (1) the patient has worked through the problem already, or (2) the patient has repressed it or dissociated from it severely, and the abreactive work has not even begun.

Not every instance of sexual trauma will lead to pseudoseizures. On the basis of my clinical experience, I have identified two factors which are likely to predispose the patient to the development of psychogenic spells. These are (1) the state of cognitive inconsistency or dissonance and (2) pathology of parental communication with the child.

Cognitive dissonance is a concept developed by Festinger (1957), who hypothesized that human beings seek to keep their ideas about the world and about themselves in a state of harmony or balance. Notions that are incompatible with one another cause tension and discomfort. With regard to the issue of trauma, the patient whose trauma is of such a nature as to cause him or her to be in a psychologically untenable or intolerable situation is more likely to react poorly, and be more vulnerable to the development of pseudoseizure (or other somatizing coping styles). For example, if the perpetrator of the trauma is a person with whom the patient otherwise has a relationship, and especially if that person has made her feel worthy or special, so that the feeling between the two is not just or even predominantly animosity, this type of situation is likely to generate cognitive inconsistency. For example, the patient may wonder: "How can someone who hurt me and humiliated me, be someone who loved me or made me feel special?" Or, "How can I still care or have cared about someone who caused me such pain?" Incest is particularly likely to place the patient in a psychologically untenable position for obvious reasons, in that it involves a relationship or behavior that is not sanctioned, and until very recently could not even be discussed.

Patients who have survived motor vehicle accidents may also struggle with marked cognitive inconsistencies, especially if the accident occurred through no fault of their own. The patient may experience intense anger at the person who caused the accident and all the difficulties that followed but did not offer any restitution. It should be pointed out that even those accidents that do not leave obvious lesions or that cause only minimal CNS damage can nonetheless substantially disrupt the patient's life. For example, establishing whether or not the spells that develop after the accident are epileptic may, in itself, take a considerable period of time. Thus, the situation in which the patient finds himself can stimulate intense anger, which the patient is, in a sense, stuck with, because no one can reverse the events as they occurred.

In such circumstances, one may encounter persistent displacement of anger onto professionals, or the development of psychogenic spells as a defense against anger (dissociative defense). Nightmares or night terrors may be yet another method of shunting the anger and protecting the patient's ego from being overwhelmed.

The pathology of parental communication is another factor that is especially significant in the development of pseudoseizures. Patients with traumatic pseudoseizures often report that their parents communicated with them in ways that appear quite pathological; the outcome of which was to ignore, deny, or distort the child's experience of the world, or his/her own body. It is well known that a part of the parental role is to validate the child's experience of reality, and to support his perceptions and feelings, so that the child may eventually grow to rely on his own feelings and perceptions as the natural starting point in his approach to life. If the parents fail to provide this essential validation because they are narcissistic, pathologically rigid, or too invested in being infallible, such that what the child says is treated as irrelevant, the child may learn that his or her feelings or judgments of reality are of no value, and cannot be relied on to get through life.

The pathological communication on the part of parents may take different forms. Some parents, while not neglectful of other areas of a child's life, may exhibit a stony indifference with regard to the child's emotions, physical experiences, or interpretations of reality. For them, the child's feelings have no reality as such. Later on in life, the patient is similarly estranged from his own feelings: "I felt something very strongly, but there was no substance to what I was feeling." Other parents are inclined to magical thinking. Their reality testing is dominated by their needs, and they have a very fluid and loose approach to reality testing. One patient, for example, recalled being told that her favorite sister died because the patient forgot to tell her that she loved her.

Parents described in these two categories are perceived by the child as damaging and hurtful. There is a third group of parents who do not intend to be either damaging or hurtful, but are instead inadequate and cannot cope with the child's feelings (nor perhaps with their own). The parent cannot successfully articulate either positive or negative feelings. This type of parent, often the mother, may be caring in other ways, but is quite deficient in the role of one who validates the child's feelings. She is difficult for the child to cope with because the child, while sensing that the mother is failing in some important way, cannot readily identify why she is failing and cannot get angry at her because she is not perceived as hurtful or hostile.

Yet another group of patients with pseudoseizures who frequently report pathology of parental communication are adult children of alcoholics. As children, they are faced with a raging and unreasonable parent (often the father). One method of adapting to a parent who is out of control is to seek effortfully to develop a solid structure in one's own life, and to be conscientious, dutiful, productive, and most importantly to focus on solving problems, and not on interpreting feelings. This line of adaptation can lead to substantial, even superior, achievement. However, the person is at the same time burdened by a fear of the humiliating chaos into which the family was plunged (due to the parent's alcoholism), which the child seeks to avoid at all costs. Along with the child's desire to be very dutiful and to control things in very careful ways, there is also a parallel fear of emotional experience. This does not include only negative feelings, but any emotional experience as such. Feelings are feared intrinsically because they can mobilize frightening memories of chaos and a raging parent. The adult child of an alcoholic parent may find it virtually impossible to separate emotions from chaos.

Thus, the various forms of pathological communication reviewed above tend to generate mistrust in the patient of his or her own feelings and judgment. This estrangement from one's own experience can render a person vulnerable to somatization for the simple reason that the person has never learned how to express feelings in words or has been actively discouraged from doing so by parental interference and distortion. It is easy to see how a person so ill-equipped to read feelings and make them understandable to others would be especially disadvantaged if he or she suffered a trauma. Having to process a painful and complex situation without being able to recognize and interpret feelings may make the person especially vulnerable to developing somatizing or dissociative states.

Trauma due to head injury or postconcussive state

This occurs in patients with postconcussive syndrome, especially males, who also suffer from PTSD as a result of a motor vehicle accident. The post-traumatic component in many victims of motor vehicle accidents is often neglected; yet, it exacerbates the postconcussive state considerably. Indeed, it is this combination of postconcussive and PTSD symptomatology which makes the syndrome so challenging for the patient to tolerate, and for the clinicians to fully understand and treat.

Traumatic head injury can affect one's emotional and personality functioning in a variety of ways. The clinical picture is thus often richly symptomatic. In a recent review of literature, Prigatano (1992), who has distinguished himself by his studies of head-injured patients and has written about their emotional difficulties extensively, lists a variety of symptoms. These include irritability, agitation, anger, emotional liability and rapid mood changes, aspontaneity and loss of interest in the environment, depression, anxiety, and the catastrophic reaction and unawareness of deficits. While patients with pseudoseizures due to head injury in our category include those with less CNS impairment than those considered by Prigatano, the symptomatology listed by Prigatano provides a very useful framework for understanding our own cases.

As is well known, motor vehicle accidents often involve numerous traumatic experiences, feelings of terror, physical trauma or injury, threat of loss of life, neuropsychological deficits (typically attention and memory), financial losses, limitations in work performance, loss of status, and the necessity of consulting numerous physicians. In addition to well-delineated and well-understood sequelae, motor vehicle accidents often, in my experience, present with vague and shifting sensations and experiences that are difficult for the patient to understand and describe, both to himself and to others.

The patient is not merely dealing with a specific deficit, but rather, with a situation in which his experience of himself is, overall, somewhat different than before, as though it has shifted. This sense of things being somehow shifted, in addition to numerous other problems and deficits, changes the patient's experience in a comprehensive, not discrete, way, which is very difficult to integrate emotionally. Second, some deficits or various poorly defined sensations are quite variable and change from day to day. This places the patient in a dilemma when he tries to explain to himself and others something that does not stay the same from day to day. A useful metaphor for viewing the postconcussive/posttraumatic symptoms picture is to imagine a cauldron in which something is bubbling all the time, but not in the same place twice.

Finally, various sensations and deficits are difficult to define and articulate. Prigatano has commented on the patients' lack of awareness of their deficits, which is, in its own right, a deficit (Prigatano, 1992). I am inclined to take this point even further by proposing that some deficits and changes in the overall body experience are inherently difficult to verbalize because they are difficult to conceptualize in the first place. We simply do not have words to describe how things are not the same. This is because the experiences of sameness, wholeness, and normalcy are so embedded in the foundations of identity that we do not think of them as separate functions. They are so extremely fundamental that we lack terms to describe them.

Another point worth considering has to do with the blurring of the boundaries between cognitive and emotional phenomena. In the patient's actual experience these phenomena are typically blended, as indeed they are in noninjured people. For the sake of scientific and clinical investigation we categorized the sequelae of head injury into emotional and cognitive, and this distinction has an obvious heuristic value. However, this distinction is less useful when we try to understand the patient's subjective (that is, actual) experience. For example, concentration and memory are typically considered as cognitive functions par excellence. Yet, concentration can also be thought of as that function which underlies our engagement with the environment (and ourselves) and permits us to derive meaning from it. Memory, on the other hand, links the ongoing with the previous experience and enables us to perceive the continuity of experience. Thus, concentration and memory mediate our capacity to both derive meaning and to ensure the continuity of meaning. In that sense, they are the very foundations of our sense of self and our sense of continuity of self through time, namely, identity. Having variable and unpredictable concentration and attention (notoriously common in this population) means that patients cannot remain involved with the environment long enough to derive meaning from things. Things previously taken for granted, such as reading an article in one sitting, now become laborious and painstaking and require maximal effort for minimal return. This alters one's entire basis for evaluating oneself. Not being able to remember means that one cannot have confidence in what one knows (Did something happen or not?). This means that one cannot be certain that one is in touch with reality, which presents a very significant emotional problem as well.

In sum, the patient may have difficulty interpreting (tagging, or labeling) what is happening to him. It is obvious then that he will have even more difficulty making his complaints clear to others. Even when the patient can do this, other people (clinicians and family) may have difficulty understanding the complaint, which means they will certainly have difficulty validating and accepting it. This happens because the complaint, being poorly understood by the patient, is described vaguely or in metaphoric terms, tending to raise suspicions of psychiatric illness. The problem the patient has in making himself understood is made even more difficult if he has only mild or minimal CNS impairment (according to imaging studies) and no physical injury. In that situation, there is a marked discrepancy between the patient's perception of the severity of damage and adverse change and the perceptions of family and clinicians. This discrepancy makes the patient vulnerable to being considered a malingerer. Thus, an impasse can develop in which both parties are challenged by one another. This impasse can be overcome if one acknowledges that it is no one's fault, and that the syndrome entails many unpredictable changes that are difficult for all concerned to characterize and deal with.

Thus, the postconcussive male may need to face numerous limitations, the sum total of which can affect his functioning in almost all dimensions of independent living. These in turn are precisely those dimensions that define the adult male in our culture. Thus, the sum total of what we term *sequelae of head injury* may amount to having to reinvent one's life, rather than having to just deal with a disorder. This, in turn, requires a great willingness to accept the losses and narcissistic injuries without undue rage or acting out or, on the other hand, without becoming unduly dependent on one's spouse. It demands willingness to invest in the world again, and to be ready to actively seek to develop new terms by which to live one's life. These are formidable tasks, which are, nonetheless, implicitly asked of the patient when others expect him to get better.

In my own work, I have observed that postconcussive males who develop pseudoseizures tend to cluster in a very narrow age range: mid-30s to 40 years old. This is the period of midlife crisis (or immediately preceding it) or midlife review.

According to Levinson (1977), who has studied adult male development, this period of mid-30s and early 40s involves two closely related stages, each with its specific psychological requirement. The earlier stage requires that one consolidate one's position with regard to major life tasks, "establish a niche in society and become a valued member of a valued world" (Levinson, 1977). This phase thus involves solidifying one's commitments. The stage that follows, which occurs around the age of 40, involves reevaluating those commitments and reassessing their continued value in one's life (Levinson, 1977).

A postconcussive male may find it particularly difficult to cope successfully with requirements of both stages. At a time when others are using their skills maximally and making the most of their opportunities to achieve success, the patient must learn to live with his limitations and change his aspirations, whether he wishes to or not. Feelings of envy and resentment may arise over the intrinsic injustice of having been in an accident and being set back. These feelings are a legitimate part of the post-traumatic grieving process and are not due to a character disorder or a desire for compensation. The patient is faced with the necessity of somehow working through these feelings without even being comfortable acknowledging them. In addition, adjustment to head trauma (even a mild one) may lead to changes in the patient's marital relationship. The patient typically recedes into a more passive and demanding role, whereas the spouse tends to assume, increasingly, the complementary role of a caretaker (rather than a partner). Thus the patient and his (her) spouse, while still in their 30s or early 40s, may be forced to deal with issues that are very similar to issues found in aged couples.

In view of the sheer number, as well as severity, of challenges that face patients in this category, it is not surprising that they may develop pseudoseizures as a means of escaping a massive psychological threat that cannot be handled in any simple or immediate way.

Chronic traumatic life course

This is a distinct subset of the PTPS most commonly seen in females in their late thirties or early forties. Trauma plays a very significant role here as well, although it is not so much a single trauma as a chronically traumatic and challenging lifestyle. Such patients often present with histories marked by hardships, poverty, or marginal financial circumstances necessitating constant struggle. In addition, their histories often include multiple marriages, often to partners with significant difficulties of their own (such as substance abuse) or partners who may be physically abusive. Often, such patients have not received adequate nurturance in their family of origin and learned, instead, to take care of others as a means of maintaining relationships. Often, they are single parents without much support. There may be concurrent or past history of epilepsy.

Pseudoseizures may be diagnosed with some delay, and after much professional effort, because the patient may present with many different types of spells, or spells that occur in conjunction with migraines or anxiety states. In spite of their traumatic lives and many losses, such women, in my experience, tend to be, or can be, very strong and resilient. In a word, they are survivors, rather than the reverse. They learned to cope with external circumstances and stressors, but may neglect (or have never learned to attend to) their feelings, and do not process the impact of all the adverse events on their lives. Thus, a substantial lag develops between coping with external problems and coping with emotions. The latter lags significantly behind.

This style of coping is understandable in circumstances in which there are few material resources and few people who care and will help. In such a context, one may not be able to afford to focus on feelings a good deal because there are constantly pressing existential problems. The lag between external coping and emotional processing makes the patient vulnerable to the development of psychogenic spells. It is interesting that these spells tend to develop after the patient's life has stabilized, at least to some extent, and the patient is in a more favorable life situation. Thus, there may be a considerable delay, often of many years', between the end of the most intensely difficult period in the patients' lives and the development of psychogenic spells. This lack of apparent connection often puzzles both the patient and the clinicians treating them. The reason for the lag or the delay lies in the fact that emotional issues cannot be indefinitely suppressed and ignored. Their surfacing may be further prompted by the occurrence of additional psychological stressors, such as midlife concerns and crises that force one to review one's life and face unresolved issues.

Developmental pseudoseizure syndrome

In this category, pseudoseizures are thought to result not from a single trauma, or even a chronically traumatic life course, but rather, from a difficulty coping with major and complex life tasks of psychosocial development. The term *developmental* does not mean that pseudoseizure syndrome develops gradually; but rather, it refers specifically to psychosocial development. A typical clinical picture is of a patient with chronic epilepsy, often present since childhood, whose seizures have come under control. It should be emphasized that patients in this category represent a specific subset of patients with chronic epilepsy, namely those with a difficult course and significant limitations. The paradigmatic case is a patient in his late 30s or even early 40s, although this can occur in patients in their 20s in similar circumstances. The patient, after a chronic illness and prolonged dependency on parents, needs to establish himself along major dimensions of independent living, such as employment and establishment of relationships. The necessity of facing these complex challenges (which are a source of difficulty even under favorable circumstances) has been postponed for many years because of a long illness. Becoming free of seizures is often interpreted as meaning that there is now no longer any legitimate reason for not achieving those adult milestones.

This assumption is, in my view, quite unrealistic; yet, it is often shared implicitly by the patient, his family and friends, and to some extent, by the treatment milieu. This may be due to a considerable discrepancy that exists between the impressive rate of progress in treating seizures themselves and the more modest rate of progress in our understanding of the psychosocial aspects of chronic epilepsy. It is true that epilepsy is well known as a disorder that can cause considerable psychological difficulties. It is also true that psychopathology of epilepsy continues to be studied. However, much of that research has focused on symptomatic disturbances or well-delineated clinical entities, such as anxiety disorders, affective disorders, character disorder, and psychoses. This approach is certainly useful and obviously necessary to establish the parameters of the problem. However, much less attention has been devoted to understanding the impact of epilepsy on psychosocial development and, particularly, the development of object relations. Yet, clinical experience clearly demonstrates that many difficult conditions are not symptomatic disturbances, but stem from more fundamental deficits in ego development. Prolonged illness and dependency often interfere with various tasks of psychosocial development and maturity, especially in epilepsy where one is not only dealing with illness, but specifically with numerous and unpredictable changes in the level and nature of awareness that seizures cause. While it is true that individual differences may be striking, it is prudent to consider that the patient may have missed opportunities for some types of social learning necessary for ego development, which may make it more difficult for him/her to function interpersonally. Yet, the specific nature of those deficits remains poorly understood.

These, and related issues, need to be considered because major attainments of adulthood, such as maintaining employment and marriage or stable relationships, are built precisely on the foundations of earlier psychological milestones.

In addition to the possibility of not having completed successfully some stages of psychosocial development, the patients in this group are also struggling with the ambivalence regarding separation from the parents, typically the mother. In many instances, one encounters a mother/adult child dyad, which functions as a well-integrated system that has evolved over a long period of time. Both the adult son and the mother are facing a developmental challenge of a new stage. The patient, in his late 30s or early 40s, is facing the necessity of separating and establishing independence, which is essentially the task of young adulthood. However, this is occurring at a stage that is normatively associated with midlife review. Thus, he may be experiencing not only a challenge of one stage, but of the demands of one stage conflicting with the demands of another, later stage.

The ambivalence over separating from the parent can be quite intense, and it may involve guilt concerning independence and also various irrational, but keenly felt, anxieties, such as the dread of relying on one's own judgment and acting on the basis of one's own feelings. Also, the possibility that the parent might be aging and becoming weaker may stimulate a fear in the patient that he will become weak as well. This occurs because the issues of separation/individuation, particularly the rapprochement phase (Mahler, 1972), can be quite pronounced, especially the difficulty in knowing how one's own feelings or states are different from those of a parent. These, and similar anxieties, are very difficult to define and verbalize, and the patient may not be able to readily articulate them in therapy. They are not immediately apparent in social circumstances, but only become felt in close ties.

The parent, on the other hand, has equally difficult challenges to face. In my experience, the caretaking parent is typically the mother who has, in many instances, devoted decades of her life to caring for the patient and has demonstrated remarkable persistence and commitment. Her child is, in a very real sense, her life's work. It is interesting to note, in this context, that while these instances of remarkable dedication to a sick child well into adulthood are, in my experience, very common, they are rarely acknowledged as anything special. Frequently, they are simply taken for granted as being a part of the maternal role. Considering that the care of patients with a chronic illness such as epilepsy requires skills that go well beyond the average, expectable parental responsibilities, this lack of social recognition or even symbolic reward is quite extraordinary. Developmentally, the aging mother, now in her 60s, is herself in a period of transition. Studies of adult development and aging show that males and females undergo a reversal of their usual roles in the latter part of life (Jung, 1933, quoted in Gutmann, 1987). Males, whose traditional roles require them to be assertive, independent, and oriented toward problem solving (instrumental orientation), may, in later years, evolve qualities of greater nurturance and may become more accepting of their own dependency needs. Women, on the other hand, follow the opposite trajectory from a nurturant, supportive orientation toward greater assertiveness and active mastery of the environment (Gutmann, 1987).

In discussing these changes, one needs to bear in mind that one is not necessarily dealing with dramatic behavioral changes, but rather with changes in personality organization and relative emphases on the "masculine" versus "feminine" psychological potentials within the individual (Gutmann, 1987).

One of the possible changes in the feminine role in later years has to do with the "lessening of the parental imperative" (Gutmann, 1987). This means that there may be a tendency for the parent to be less intensely involved in the parental commitments on a day-to-day basis. How this stage-related pressure for change affects the aging mother of a patient with chronic epilepsy is still poorly understood. Is the mother, for example, able to disengage, even to a small extent, from the very sustained commitment and nurturance without feeling anxious and guilt-ridden? Again, our knowledge of these and similar issues pertaining to the impact of epilepsy on meeting stage-related challenges by both the patient and his parents is scanty.

It is evident, however, that both partners in the dyad are faced with a frustrating dilemma. I would summarize their situation as one in which both partners wish to separate, and both wish to retain the status quo. Given the complexity of the issues, it is not difficult to imagine why pseudoseizures would provide a solution of sorts to this very involved interpersonal and emotional situation, and a means of avoiding issues that pose a massive threat.

Treatment of pseudoseizure syndromes

General treatment considerations

In undertaking treatment of patients with pseudoseizures, the same general principle should be followed that applies to any other out-patient treatment. Namely, the choice of method and technique are determined by the adequacy of the patient's ego structure and the patient's level of development in terms of object relations. These are the key dimensions determining the treatment method. This translates into a question of whether the patient is fundamentally organized on the neurotic level, as opposed to an earlier and more primitive (borderline, narcissistic) level of development. The nature of symptoms should obviously be considered. However, the same symptom may have different significance, which calls for a different intervention based on the level of the patient's ego organization. For example, persistent depressive states in a neurotic patient have a different meaning than estrangement and depletion of a narcissistic patient. Thus, the stability and robustness of the patient's overall coping determines the choice of treatment interventions or a relative emphasis on interpretation versus support and education.

Post-traumatic pseudoseizure syndrome

Psychodynamic psychotherapy

My treatment of choice is psychodynamic psychotherapy, which contains a combination of treatment strategies appropriate for oedipal, as well as pre-oedipal, levels of personality organization. Psychodynamic therapy with this group contains the following important areas of emphasis or treatment agenda.

Reconceptualization of the nature of pseudoseizures

Pseudoseizures are often perceived, both by the patients and their families, as something that occurs to the patient, and is visited upon them from some external source and for some obscure reason, which has very little to do with who they are psychologically and how they deal with their lives. Not uncommonly, the patient is seen as a passive victim of a bizarre condition. In sum, pseudoseizures are conceptualized as something the patient *has* as opposed to something he *does*. This fallacy was recognized, and its implications elaborated by behavioral psychologists. The corollary of this basic assumption is that someone else, namely, the neurologist or a psychologist, will rid them of this condition, and that it is the clinician's responsibility to eliminate this problem (and not the patient's). A further assumption is that success of therapy is defined as a reduction in the number of spells. Obviously, these three assumptions are not only erroneous, but they represent major stumbling blocks in the treatment of patients with clearly psychogenic spells. Therapy consists of helping the patient realize, in a gradual and reasonable way, that spells are something the patient does in order to deal with something that disturbs him (that is, spells have a purpose in his life). Thus, therapy entails a major conceptual shift in the patient's attitude toward the pseudoseizures; it is a shift away from being seen as a strange condition afflicting a passive victim, toward a more productive view of pseudoseizures as signs of difficulty coping with a problem. Pseudoseizures are thus reformulated from being a sign of disease to being a sign of a problem in coping. The patients who accomplish this shift have traversed a major milestone, making all other exploration possible. Being able to traverse this milestone is, in its own right, a strong positive prognostic sign. On the other hand, patients who continue to insist on symptomatic relief alone, and continue to view their spells as having nothing to do with them psychologically, have a poor prognosis; their reaction amounts to the rejection of exploring the cause of their problem. However, this is relatively rare; it is more likely to occur much earlier, at the stage at which the patient is first informed that his/her spells are pseudoseizures and is struggling to decide whether to enter therapy or not. The resistance to the idea of psychological causation can persist for months, and it should not be viewed too pessimistically, as long as the patient remains in therapy and is engaged in it, in spite of this resistance. This issue requires time to resolve.

In this context, it may be appropriate to comment further on the issue of symptomatic relief. In my experience, symptomatic relief is both possible and desirable. However, defining it as a goal of treatment carries risk. First, it is difficult to treat pseudoseizures directly, and it is impossible to offer guarantees that psychological treatment will eliminate them. Second, in view of the post-traumatic nature of a sizable proportion of pseudoseizure cases, I consider it important to uncover the trauma, or at least bear the possibility of a trauma in mind, since the emotional cost of an untreated post- traumatic state is high. Even when the origin of pseudoseizure is not clearly post-traumatic, but is related to some other emotional issue, it is very important to be able to identify this issue and treat it.

The pacing function of the therapist

In patients with pseudoseizures, particularly those who rely heavily on suppression, repression, denial, and dissociation, there is a tendency to deal with experience as a whole, as opposed to dealing with it in a gradual and piecemeal way. The patients behave as if they believed that there were only two ways of dealing with their emotional experience (especially traumatic): (1) to avoid or suppress it totally or (2) to feel it in its entirety and be overwhelmed by it (absorb it, or eject it). This is related to the so-called *bi-phasic* mode of handling emotion, which is well known in post-traumatic states in general (Van der Kolk and Ducey, 1989). In a sense, the patient acts as if once she begins to feel or remember past feelings, she will not be able to stop and will lose control or lose her sanity. The patients rarely verbalize that fear, however, and may seem embarrassed when it is interpreted. A related assumption is that, just as their spells are sudden and paroxysmal, so should the relief and resolution occur in a similarly sudden and absolute manner (also rarely recognized by the patient).

The therapist can be very helpful by educating patients as to the fact that recovery from difficult feelings and issues is a gradual process, and that they can proceed at a pace that is *tolerable* (important word) to them. Furthermore, I tend to add that in this process, their mind (may use term "unconscious") will assist us, and will provide material according to its own schedule, and according to the patient's ability to handle it. Dreams may also help. This intervention permits the patient to tolerate difficult material better, since it is presented as providing needed information. This is an important point in treatment of pseudoseizure patients or those patients who dissociate or are, for various reasons, terrified by their feelings and see their mind as a source of strange troubles and symptoms. This estrangement can be bridged if their unconscious mind is reconceptualized as an ally. In sum, I encourage the patient to assume responsibility for setting the pace and for reporting promptly if the feelings evoked are intolerable. Again, this may seem an obvious point. However, in my work with this group of patients, I have discovered that they frequently harbor fears that the therapist will lead them into experiencing intolerable feelings and then leave them to struggle alone.

A part of the pacing function of the therapist is to manage the abreactive episodes which occur in sessions. In those cases, pseudoseizures are a part of the abreactive episode. These episodes are quite distinctive and easy to recognize. They often begin with a change in the quality of the patient's voice, usually a regression to a child's voice (dissociative aspect). This is followed by pseudoconvulsive posturing, which may involve sliding to the floor and crouching in the corner, crying "Don't hurt me!" Sometimes, the patient's verbalizations are unintelligible, or the patient slurs his/her words. These episodes are self-limiting, and in my experience, do not involve injury. Upon recovery, I treat these episodes as I do any other event in therapy that has information value. I ask the patient how they are feeling (doing), and I also ask them to tell me what they are experiencing. I do not treat the event as being special. Indeed, a matter-of-fact, but concerned approach works best, a point also made by McDade and Brown (1992) in their discussion of management of pseudoseizures in an in-patient setting. Dramatizing the event or treating it with undue significance reinforces the wrong assumption that we should focus on the spell, rather than on the patient.

Recovery of experience

In our earlier discussion of the post-traumatic symptomatology, we commented on the restriction of emotional experience and the impoverishment of emotional expression. This traumatic loss of ability to experience (and also to recognize different experiences) is one of the most significant aspects of chronic PTSD. Consequently, the recovery of the ability to experience emotion, and to experience a wider range of feelings, are the most important therapeutic tasks with patients with PTPS.

This task is not limited to emotions, but extends to the patient's perceptions and judgments of reality, as well as their willingness to take initiative. Due to a combination of trauma and the pathology of parental communication, which teaches patients to mistrust their own judgment, they may now show a marked reluctance to rely on their own interpretation of their environment and whatever is happening in their own bodies. Those pseudoseizure patients who also have a history of epilepsy since childhood are especially likely to mistrust their experience because they have often suffered from unpredictable fluctuations in the level of awareness, which can obviously undermine their faith in what they know. Further problems occur when the family attributes the patient's perceptions to side effects of medications, or worse yet, when the patient's experience is dismissed altogether by such statements as "That never happened, you had a seizure and imagined it."

A pseudoseizure patient's lack of trust in her own judgment is not immediately apparent. Indeed, it only becomes apparent after painstaking efforts to explore many "pseudo-issues". For example, the patient may have a conventional dilemma between asserting her independence as an adult (vis-a-vis parents) and allowing her parents to interpret her feelings for her or tell her what to do. The patient may bring this issue up over and over again. On the surface, this resembles a process aimed at problem solving. It really is not because the outcome is always the same, namely no option works and the patient is immobilized, suggesting there is no solution. In fact, the patient is not seeking a solution, but is seeking a way of not having to rely on her own perceptions and judgments, namely, avoiding knowing what she actually knows. A related fear is having to act upon one's perceptions and feelings. The act of relying on one's own feelings is intrinsically threatening and is feared in its own right, and not because the patient's judgment might be inadequate. A clue that this process might be at work is an undue preoccupation on the patient's part with finding the best approach to the problem, not merely an approach. This superficially resembles perfectionism, but is not. In such situations, I have found it useful to say something like this: "I am less concerned with whether you will handle the situation well. It is more important that we know what you feel in the first place. Once we do, you will handle the situation in a way you see fit." At this point, the patient may say "But how do I act before all this is clear to me?" I have found that giving the patient permission to "muddle along" (because this is a legitimate manner of acting when one is uncertain) tends to bring surprising relief, especially if the therapist is comfortable with humor and metaphor in general.

This type of intervention communicates several points. First, it emphasizes that one's own feelings are the natural starting point of any decision. Second, it communicates to the patient that his/her approach to a given situation is ultimately his or her own responsibility, not the therapist's. It also "de-catastrophizes" the process of decision making by suggesting that there is no magical correct way, but that the patient will do what is possible and what seems reasonable.

Validation of the patient's experience may take many forms. One has to do with helping the patient realize that it is acceptable to have conflicts and uncertainty because one may have conflicting motivations that, although opposite, are both quite justifiable. In a way, this amounts to educating the patient that he or she has an honest conflict, not a bizarre illness. The patients in this group frequently experience shame of not just their unacceptable feelings, but also of having a feeling in general, or of being unassertive, or having doubts, and especially of having needs. In response to shame over these experiences, the patient may rapidly withdraw, disengage, or become dysphoric. Thus, the shame is rarely expressed directly, but is instead often disguised as a shift in mood. The therapist is faced with a three-fold task: (1) to uncover the original feeling, (2) to identify the patient's anxiety or shame over having that feeling, and finally, (3) to teach the patient that both are acceptable.

The patient may thus experience a conflict, a shame over being conflicted, and anger over being ashamed in very rapid succession, with these three distinct issues all blended and enmeshed. What the therapist sees, however, is not very distinct, and the patient's feeling state may be difficult to distinguish from misery. The therapist can infer that several feeling states are present from subtle, but repetitive, shifts in mood that occur in a number of related situations.

Special issues in treatment of sexual abuse survivors

The victim's bind

The victim's bind refers to a paradoxical situation in which the victim is torn between two intensely opposed motivations: (1) to forgive and forget, heal, and make a success of her life and (2) to hold on to the hurt. The victims may feel compelled to cling to the hurt because letting go of it is perceived as a form of disloyalty to their past suffering or even a form of betrayal of a part of themselves. To be content and productive again is interpreted as letting the abuser win in the end or denying what one has suffered. Davies and Frawley (1991) described this dynamic very extensively in their discussion of sexual abuse victims who develop dissociative states. A very similar dilemma was described by Krystal in his discussion of concentration camp survivors who cannot let go and accept what happened because the acceptance is experienced as "submission to persecution" (Krystal, 1981).

I would add that the victim's compulsion to cling to the trauma may be related to the unique circumstances of both sexual abuse and the concentration camp situation. In both of those circumstances, abuse occurred with complicity of others, or at least was permitted to occur by others who were indifferent. In short, the trauma victim typically did not receive (until much later) the usual human response, which is implicitly given for other kinds of suffering. Trying to preserve the pain and bear witness to it may represent, for the patients, the only way they can cope with the fact that their suffering was sanctioned by others, and was even perpetrated with malignant intent.

In treatment, it is important that the therapist help the patient identify both motivations—to forget the trauma and to cling to it—and empathize with both motivations, so that the patient can acknowledge and accept them. Helping the patient realize that both of these needs are understandable and that conflict between them is inevitable is therapeutic. In dealing with this difficult issue it is certainly important for the therapist to ally himself with the patient's life-affirming and growth-seeking self. Healing cannot occur otherwise. However, the patient should know that it is ultimately their existential right to choose whether and how much to forgive.

I should further add that the dynamics of the victim's bind do not occur with the same intensity in every case. However, it is useful to consider that this process might be the root of the problem in circumstances in which the patient is acutely agitated, unstable, or persistently suicidal.

Role of maternal deprivation (the double loss)

Sexual abuse in childhood is traumatic not only because of the obvious hurt inflicted by the abusive parent but, in many instances, because of the lack of support and compassion from the nonabusive parent. The role of the mother in abusive families is controversial, and our knowledge of this difficult problem is still evolving. However, there are several lines of evidence that suggest difficulties in early mother–child interactions. Gabbard (1991), in his discussion of patients sexually abused as children, commented on the "uninvolved mother" and maternal deprivation. He emphasized the importance of maternal deprivation in generating states of "melancholic emptiness" or "deadness". In sum, in certain instances of child sexual abuse (especially severe trauma cases) there are several layers of trauma. The first is maternal deprivation or empathic failure, which predisposes the patient to persistent anhedonia and depressiveness or even dissociative states. The second layer of trauma is the abuse itself. In a paradoxical way, the relationship with the abusive father (in its real or internalized form) may serve to protect the patient from the emptiness of the relationship with the mother (Gabbard, 1991).

In treatment, the process of remembering and abreacting the abuse may require that the patient face and work through two separate challenges. The first is coming to terms with the abuse. This entails not just coming to terms with the anger toward the father, but also sadness over the loss of a good father (which abuse implies). Second, the patient is faced with early maternal deprivation and maternal inadequacy. This amounts to mourning for *two losses*, which is a formidable task. The awareness of the lack of nurturance by the mother is something the child is especially eager to suppress/repress to survive as a person. Having to acknowledge this painful deficit as an adult can trigger powerful fears of becoming overwhelmingly depressed.

My clinical experience suggests that the above difficulties notwithstanding, the adult survivor does not wish to completely reject either parent, even the abusive parent. Indeed, one of the most powerful motivations for not disclosing the abuse is the fear of rejection by the family. The patient may feel that disclosure will destroy both the family and herself (namely, catastrophic abandonment and annihilation fantasies). In a sense, fear of confronting the family is yoked to the fear of catastrophic abandonment.

Reluctance to give up parents

In the course of therapy, the patient's feelings may alternate rapidly and unpredictably between an intense anger at the abuser on the one hand and the fear of complete loss on the other. This can be very frustrating and confusing to the patient. Again, it is important for the therapist to acknowledge and validate both sides of the ambivalence, and to help the patient realize that both anger and the desire to protect the parents are legitimate motivations.

The patients, thus, often seek to retain some kind of a bond with the parent(s), and salvage what is salvageable from the relationship. This may amount to having to develop the relationship on different terms or in a more limited way. Yet, the ability to rescue positive meaning from the relationship, even in a subtle way, can be of great importance to the patient's well-being.

Consequently, it is important that the therapist support the patient in this effort. Sometimes, the patient feels guilty for wishing to forgive the parent and maintain the relationship. She may even feel ashamed of this motivation and, not uncommonly, become intensely angry with herself for having such feelings. The anger at herself and shame are rarely explicitly acknowledged, however, and may be inferred when the patient seems "stuck" and intensely helpless or resentful. At such times the therapist can be useful to the patient by pointing out that the desire to forgive the parent (abuser) and preserve the relationship is a positive motivation and a part of their need to grow and regain control of her life.

The motivation to reject can alternate with the desire to rescue the relationship with the abuser in a very intense manner, which the patient may interpret as a lack of progress. Again, it is important that the patient be reassured that this seeming chaos is typical of the manner in which resolution of this conflict occurs. One can further comment that the patient is trying to accomplish nothing less than to re-create a new relationship with the parent—a process that is, by its very nature, characterized by trial and error.

Trauma due to head injury

In the discussion of the nature of difficulties facing a patient with pseudoseizures secondary to a motor vehicle accident, we identified three features that are especially difficult for the patient to tolerate. These have to do with the experience being changed in a comprehensive (not limited) way, the various complaints and sensations being intrinsically difficult to define and articulate, and the complaints being variable. In my experience, these difficulties are likely to stimulate a fear of fragmentation and loss of integrity of the self in the patient.

In a somewhat over-simplified way, we could say that for the neurotic patients, the main psychological threat stems from their unacceptable impulses or unconscious fantasies, whereas for the patients with CNS impairment (even mild impairment), the main threat stems from the possibility of inner disorganization. This may also include a fear of not being able to contain what one feels or even of depersonalizing. The patient experiences things that threaten his sense of sameness. The underlying fear, thus has to do with losing the sense of continuity of one's body and one's experience of the environment. The body does not feel quite the same and neither does the outside world.

It should be emphasized that fears of fragmentation, or even depersonalization, are rarely expressed by the patient in explicit terms. The patient is not likely to come to therapy complaining of a fear of loss of identity or role. Indeed, I would venture to say that some of the patient's most disturbing experiences are not likely to be brought up at all, and the therapist can only access them inferentially, after pursuing many blind alleys or dealing with seemingly unrelated anxieties. The therapist who undertakes treatment of this population needs to be prepared for this.

In a sense, the therapist's task is analogous to the task of the therapist treating a borderline patient who cannot articulate his fear of loss of boundaries or loss of self, which may prompt him to acts of self-mutilation. As in the case of the postconcussive/post-traumatic patient, the underlying anxieties are far too basic to be readily verbalizable or distinguishable from anxieties stemming from other sources.

In addition to the fear of fragmentation, there are milder disturbances that are broadly related to the sense of inadequacy. One of them is a fear of multiple perspectives. Consider, for example, a patient who is being treated by multiple clinicians, each dealing with a specific aspect of the problem (this is not rare in accident victims). In therapy, the patient tends to repeatedly go over each clinician's perspective and summarize each clinician's most recent assessment, seeking to bring them all into harmony. This may, at first glance, appear to be a form of resistance: dealing with the details of the here and now instead of psychological matters. However, the somewhat driven nature of that process may alert the psychologist to the possibility that the patient is struggling to identify something that everyone agrees on, so as to have something to hold onto. This need may be pronounced even in circumstances in which there is no disagreement at all, merely natural differences in emphasis, which professionals from different fields necessarily exhibit. For the patient, however, they are not different *nuances*, they are different *things*. This fear of multiple perspectives is due to cognitive rigidity, which is a well-known and well-accepted feature of CNS impairment.

There are other fears the patient may exhibit that could also be related to cognitive limitations. For example, the patient's fear of undergoing therapy may be rooted in the fear that he may find out something he could not contain cognitively, which will, in turn, require that he reconceptualize the view of his condition again. Subtle adjustments in point of view are not easy for patients in this category, and they may think of those adjustments not as subtle shifts but as "major overhauls". The patient may fear that in the course of psychological evaluation he will lose his familiar sense of himself and of how things are and will need to reestablish order and constancy, a task that is both tedious and stressful.

The fear of having to shift one's point of view, however, may also be related to a much more obviously psychological issue, for example, a lack of trust in others. The lack of trust, in turn, may be a part of the patient's long-standing pattern (his style of relating). In dealing with resistance in therapy with this population, it is not always immediately clear whether what we term "resistance" is due to a cognitive deficit in set shifting or to an emotional issue such as a lack of trust.

There is no simple way of deciding this issue, and the answer emerges empirically through trial and error. As a general rule, it is prudent to consider that in CNS-damaged patients (even mild levels of impairment) resistance could be due to both factors. It is important to have a sense of which process is at work at a given time, because they call for different therapeutic interventions. For example, if the resistance is due to a lack of trust or to guardedness, this is interpreted and worked through as any other issue in psychodynamic therapy. If, however, one is faced with a cognitive deficit, the therapist needs to help the patient identify his fear of having to consider different or novel points of view (because this, in turn, stimulates fear of having to change things yet again). Articulating the deficit for the patient, and empathizing with the patient concerning the deficit, enables the patient to make sense of his experience, rather than, for example, becoming promptly dysphoric, angry, or resorting to somatization. The general therapeutic approach is to render the patient's experiences, especially those that are difficult to define and label, more meaningful and to validate the patient's feelings, such as they are. As we observed earlier, the accident can alienate the patient from his experience and can fragment it. The therapist seeks to achieve coherence.

Additional treatment issues

Therapy with this group of patients may assume, at times, a meandering course, with frequent repetition of the accident or some related theme. The patient may also tend to confine himself or herself a great deal to the specifics of his or her medical care, various appointments, and so forth, in the style described as alexithymia (Sifneos, Apfel-Savitz and Frankel, 1977; Nemiah, 1973), The patient may produce material that, to the psychologist, seems quasi-psychological or not psychological at all. This may stimulate a fear in the therapist that the therapy is regressing into case management.

At such times, it is useful to consider that the thematic focus is defined more flexibly in the therapy of patients in this group. Having identified a traditional psychological issue (for example, the patient's problems with authority figures owing to conflicts with the father) does not mean that the patient will stay with this issue, offer to explore it, offer affective elaboration, or even remember it in the following session. This issue may instead be embedded with somatic complaints and the review of day-to-day matters. A similar problem may arise at the very beginning of therapy when the patient may exhibit difficulty organizing himself around psychological issues. The therapist may need to spend more time searching for the focal point around which to organize therapy. It is not prudent to insist or interpret the patient's difficulty too vigorously.

Another issue that might arise is repetition. It is true that this may be a form of resistance at times. However, in patients who have sustained a concussion and are having difficulty organizing their world again, persistent repetition of the accident (or the immediate post-accident course) may serve to reinforce a limited area of certainty. While remembering those events may not be pleasant, for the patient threatened by fears of fragmentation and loss of continuity, such repetition may reestablish a sense that at least some things stay the same from day to day. In short, repetition may have an adaptive value in building a new structure and framework within which to view one's life (staking new coordinates, so to speak).

Chronic traumatic life course

The central difficulty in patients with chronic traumatic life course is their assumption that their lives are worthwhile only if they continue to deal with stresses and crises. Because they are adept at doing so, continued crisis management has become an integral part of their self-esteem. In a paradoxical way, facing crises and disasters becomes a means of regulating self-esteem. Second, managing crises (often other people's crises) is perceived by the patient as the only way they will be valued in a relationship. Finding a mate who is giving and is managing his life places a patient (initially, at least) in a situation of an executive who has lost his job. With nothing to manage, it is difficult to feel useful or worthy of affection and respect.

If the above assumptions are pointed out, the patient in this group will have difficulty acknowledging them. The therapist's chief task is to help the patient develop a belief that it is legitimate to work toward one's own goals (academic, vocational), and be rewarded for one's work. The second goal is to help the patient realize that she is worthy of affection, and that she does not need to "buy it" by prolonged and exhausting struggles in caring for partners who have chronic difficulty coping with their lives.

Developmental pseudoseizure syndrome

The aims of treatment of patients in this category are not as easy to identify, as is the case with post-traumatic patients. This is due to the fact that delays and deficits in psychosocial development in this group are not clearly understood and can only be fully established in the course of treatment. In general, the therapist's aim is to identify whatever issues are possible for the patient to work with and to organize therapy around those. This in no way implies that psychotherapy does not work. Indeed, it can be helpful in a variety of ways. However, treatment focus needs to be established more gradually.

An important aspect of treatment of patients in this category is making treatment available to their parents, or to anyone in the family who wishes it. This especially pertains to the treatment of the mother who is, in most instances, the primary caretaker. The care of the caretaking parent is an important, yet neglected, part of treatment since she is not seen as the identified patient. The treatment of the parents is aimed at helping them recognize the importance of their contribution to the patient's life. Furthermore, the therapist who works with the parents (different from the patient's therapist, unless otherwise indicated), should help the parents work through ambivalence about their adult child becoming more independent. Guilt feelings about letting down the burden of care and letting others help may also need to be addressed.

Note on sexuality

Disturbance of sexual function, or sexual dissatisfaction, may occur in any of the patient groups we have reviewed here. Sexual abuse, for example, may lead to a variety of sexual difficulties (Browne and Finkelhor, 1986). In my own clinical work, I was impressed by the prevalence of sexual anhedonia, as well as anxiety in connection with sexuality, in patients with traumatic pseudoseizures with a history of sexual abuse. Indeed, a persistent lack of sexual interest, in conjunction with nightmares, may be useful diagnostically in identifying patients with post-traumatic conditions.

Sexual complaints or difficulties may occur in patients with head trauma or postconcussive syndrome as well. Kosteljanetz et al. (1981) studied a group of 19 male patients with a postconcussive syndrome. They found that 53 percent of the patients reported "reduced libido", whereas erectile dysfunction was found in 42 percent of the sample. Garden, Bontke, and Hoffman (1990) studied reports of sexual functioning and satisfaction in couples in whom one of the spouses had suffered a closed head injury. They discovered that 47 percent of the couples reported dissatisfaction with their frequency of intercourse. While these studies did not deal specifically with head-injured patients who develop pseudoseizures, they provide a useful context in which to place the pseudoseizure patients with post-concussive syndrome.

Difficulties with sexual functioning have been reported in patients who suffer from epilepsy, independently of pseudo-seizures. For example, hyposexuality, or "poverty of drive", was found to be a rather common form of sexual difficulty in a sample of patients with temporal lobe epilepsy who were candidates for epilepsy surgery (Taylor, 1969). In another study that involved a group of 33 adult male outpatients with documented complex partial seizures, the author found hyposexuality in 48 percent of the sample (Pritchard, 1980). Finally, in a pilot study of 50 women with epilepsy who were treated with anticonvulsant medications at a university clinic, the authors identified a distinct sub-group who reported hyposexuality (Bergen, Daugherty and Eckenfels, 1992).

The nature and prevalence of various sexual difficulties in patients with pseudoseizures or chronic epilepsy have not been precisely established. The studies reviewed above should be viewed as descriptive and orientational, rather than as offering conclusive prevalence estimates. However, they are very useful as they underscore the importance of investigating this area of functioning (Garden, Bontke, and Hoffman, 1990), which is often neglected in routine evaluations.

Inquiry about sexual functioning should be a routine part of both a neurologist's, as well as a psychologist's evaluations. The aim of the inquiry is to identify dysfunction (especially if it is treatable), but also to enable the patient to feel comfortable discussing this area of functioning. Thus, one should not only consider frequency, or presence or absence of sexual contact, but also whether the patient derives pleasure and meaning from it. In my clinical experience, the patients are highly reluctant to bring up sexual complaints spontaneously. Yet, it is important that they be identified, especially in survivors of sexual trauma in which sexual disturbance represents an ongoing sequela of the trauma. It is also very important to be aware of it in postconcussive males in whom sexual problems may contribute to lowered self-esteem, depression, and marital stress. Thus, sensitivity to these issues is recommended and may, indeed, contribute to the quality of care.

Section II

Psychodynamics and Psychotherapy of Pseudoseizures

Introduction

In Section I, we presented a diagnostic classification scheme which permits the clinician to categorize pseudoseizures into major subtypes, each with its characteristic symptomatology and dynamic issues. This classification scheme is advantageous, because it allows the clinician to organize the clinical picture, and find his or her way amongst the complexities of pseudoseizure histories and symptomatology.

Section II represents an effort to deal with the psychodynamics of pseudoseizure syndromes in a much more intense and comprehensive way. In this work we take the view that pseudoseizures are largely post-traumatic disturbances. Post-traumatic syndromes of pseudoseizure patients are a part of a large continuum of post-traumatic syndromes of which classical PTSD (post-traumatic stress disorder) is only one variant. Pseudoseizure patients frequently present with complex, partial of chronic variants of post-traumatic disturbances.

Pseudoseizure syndromes cannot be understood in terms of a single issue or a single psychodynamical mechanism, nor can they be understood in terms of a single theory. Nor is there a unified theory of trauma which would account for all of its facets. This by no means implies that pseudoseizures/traumatic syndromes are an inert, or worse yet, a random, collection of symptoms and psychiatric diagnoses. The classification of pseudoseizure syndromes presents the first framework provided in this book for containing this complexity.

The present section is an attempt to pursue the psychodynamics further and place the observations which emerged as a result of intensive clinical inquiry into a wider context. This wider conceptual context is defined by three different schools of what can be broadly referred to as psychodynamic theory. The observations and concepts presented in this section of the book represent the second framework for understanding pseudoseizures.

We shall review the following:

Select contributions from psychoanalytic theory

In this section, we shall focus on Freud's discussion of mourning, especially complicated mourning. There are two reasons for this choice. First, complicated mourning has a role in the development of depressive symptomatology and affective symptoms are a significant part of the post-traumatic picture. Second, the mechanism of complicated morning is very relevant to the development of post-traumatic conditions. Indeed, we see it as one of the key features which characterize the psychological struggle of traumatized patients.

Complicated mourning is a great deal more than passive grief. It has a great capacity to generate conflict. The presence of conflict, in turn, complicates greatly psychological situation of the bereaved individual in such a way that the psychodynamic picture of complicated mourning begins to resemble the psychodynamic picture of someone who was traumatized.

The second important contribution has to do with the psychoanalytic concept of *internalization* of experience, particularly the internalization of loss, trauma and conflicted relationships. This mechanism helps us understand why people do not simply go through traumatic experience and get over it as a matter of course. The mechanism of internalization helps us deal with the fact that closure in traumatic conditions which come to our attention is not achieved automatically. The concept of internalization thus enables us to account for some of the complexity and chronicity which often accompany adaptation and recovery from trauma.

Select contributions from object-relations theory

A certain proportion of pseudoseizure cases regress—as a consequence of trauma—to the level of functioning characteristic of borderline syndromes, without being borderline personality disorders. Borderline phenomena represent a qualitatively different type of affect regulation and interpersonal relating.

In order to understand the nature of those phenomena it is important to review the relevant concepts from object-relations theory. Among the key concepts reviewed are particular regressive changes in the quality of affect, the pervasive need to regulate affect through other people (the need for containment), the need to get rid of negative affect through projective identification and fusional attachments.

Select contributions from self psychology

Trauma frequently leads to *narcissistic injury* and it is therefore important to recognize narcissistic injury and its key features: shame and defensive rage, as well as immobilization. Narcissistic injury figures prominently in the clinical picture of a certain proportion of traumatically based pseudoseizure syndromes. The concepts of self-cohesion (i.e., narcissistic equilibrium), and its opposite which is narcissistic vulnerability and its especially poignant acute form—narcissistic injury—were all developed in the context of self psychology.

Narcissistic injury is a particular kind of traumatic experience which has unique features and unique dynamics which need to be understood in order to be able to deal with the patient's experience. An unresolved narcissistic injury has a profound capacity to stall recovery and adaptation. It is very difficult to build on a foundation of narcissistic injury. It is likewise very difficult to mobilize the patient's psychological resources toward productive goals—even if those goals are well within their reach—if they are significantly narcissistically injured.

Unrecognized and untreated narcissistic injury can present a special problem in rehabilitation settings in which head trauma patients are treated. If the patient has reacted to head trauma primarily as a narcissistic injury, the efforts to engage him in the usual rehabilitation activities may be met with strong resistance. This resistance is a great deal more than a lack of compliance. In fact, it has nothing to do with compliance. It has to do with a sense of injured self-coherence which is, from the patient's point of view, a much more urgent psychological matter.

Understanding that it can occur and why it occurs is already an important step in approaching traumatized individuals.

Points of organization

In order to make various psychodynamic concepts meaningful, an attempt was made to bring forth enough material from each respective theory to make a particular concept feel like a natural part of a given framework. In order to achieve this important goal, a good deal of background material was presented first.

For example, in order to understand characteristic regressive changes in borderline syndromes (which pseudoseizure patients can exhibit) it is at first essential to review contributions of object-relations theory with respect to the nature of attachment. Object-relations theorists are primarily theorists of attachment, and they see the structure of personality as arising from maturational changes in the nature of attachment. They also conceptualize psychopathology as a regression to a level of affect and relatedness which belongs to an earlier stage.

In order to understand psychodynamic functions of pseudoseizures as a defense against intolerable traumatic memories, or a defense against anger elicited by a traumatic event, it is important to understand the nature of the psychodynamic mechanism of internalization, as well as the meaning of psychological defense in general. Freud's essay (1917) "Mourning and Melancholia" is valuable in this respect for two reasons. It provides a very accurate picture of the process of what is currently referred to as complicated mourning .It also provides an account of chief psychodynamic concepts in an encapsulated form. I thus presented, in some detail, the dynamics of mourning and loss, as outlined by Freud, first, and then followed it with the discussion in which its relevance to pseudoseizure cases is shown.

The concept of narcissistic injury which is a disruption in self-cohesion cannot be understood without reviewing first the processes which participate vitally in the consolidation of the sense of self. These processes involve specific favorable interactions with significant childhood figures in which the sense of self was confirmed in value.

In order to arrive at an understanding of those important mechanisms of the growth of self, I first reviewed the developmental theory of Heinz Kohut and its central concepts. Subsequently, I explored the implications of his theory for traumatic conditions and pseudoseizures.

Select contributions from psychoanalytic theory, object-relations theory and self psychology are presented in Section II of this work. Each of these three contributions is a self-contained unit and is more or less autonomous from the other two. Each unit contains theoretical background necessary for understanding the key concepts. Implications for pseudoseizure patients are presented after the relevant dynamical concept has been dealt with.

Choice of the psychodynamic mechanisms and theories

A clinician seeking to approach the material presented in this part of the book may naturally ask why these particular psychodynamic mechanisms and theories were chosen and not some others. The choice was based on that which emerged as most compelling and relevant in my work with these patients.

How should the clinician use the material to be presented? Each of the three major contributions (psychoanalytic theory, object-relations theory and self psychology) represents a somewhat different context and a different way of thinking. Each provides unique insights. The clinician is encouraged to begin by a simple question: Is the particular psychodynamic issue I have identified most like complicated mourning, or most like regression to the level of functioning characteristic of borderline syndromes, or most like narcissistic injury?

Attempting to answer the above question will provide a substantial help in organizing the dynamics of the case. Nonetheless, we should bear in mind that the patient's clinical picture may contain some aspects which can best be accounted for by psychodynamical mechanisms described under a different theoretical framework. This would not be unexpected, because, pseudoseizures syndromes are not a single entity. For his reason, we are presenting dynamic insights drawn from three separate theoretical systems.

Pseudoseizures as an ecosystem

Pseudoseizures syndromes, as well as post-traumatic syndromes, present with a great number of diverse issues and phenomena. They are, however, not a static collection of different phenomena, nor are they merely a list of symptoms (most especially not the latter).

These different phenomena do not amount to a collection in the sense that a group of paintings or apples in a basket represent a collection. Rather, they resemble parts of an ecosystem.

I propose the view that pseudoseizure syndromes, as well as traumatic syndromes, are organized as ecosystems. Different parts exist side by side and they are a part of a meaningful constellation. Yet, each component is a separate sub-system. An analogy to a garden might help illustrate how parts of an ecosystem relate to one another.

A garden is an ecosystem which exists on a track of land. Trees and birds and soil all exist in close proximity, but they are not the same thing and they are not mutually interchangeable, nor can one be translated conceptually into another. For example, the soil in the garden is a geological matter and principles and ideas which help us to understand the soil do not help us understand the migration of birds in winter. However, in order to understand the garden we need to know as much as possible about each component system, while maintaining an appreciation for the fact that the different systems still belong to the same larger ecosystem and are not side by side accidentally.

Select contributions from psychoanalytic theory

Complicated mourning and the nature of loss

In 1917, Freud published an essay entitled "Mourning and Melancholia". In this influential essay, he made important conceptual distinctions between two different types of response to loss and outlined their psychodynamic patterns.

Mourning refers to *grief,* whereas melancholia is closest to our current concept of *complicated mourning*. In this work, I take the view that complicated mourning plays a key role in a certain subset of traumatic conditions. Much of the psychological difficulty, often very disruptive and lasting, we encounter in post-traumatic states occurs as a consequence of mechanisms which occur in complicated mourning.

Both grief and complicated mourning occur in response to a loss, typically the loss of a loved one. Both involve such features as "profoundly painful dejection, abrogation of interest in the outside world, loss of the capacity to love, inhibition of all activity" (p. 153). In short, the world becomes impoverished. Complicated mourning is aggravated by the additional burden of loss of self-esteem, often very marked. This reaction is not a part of normal mourning.

The work of mourning

The process of responding to the loss of a loved one can be very intense and very laborious. One of Freud's important contributions to our understanding of depressive and post-traumatic states is his view that the person does not simply give up lost love objects as a matter of course. The process of adaptation to the loss involves an intense struggle between two strongly opposed psychological aims. On the one hand, there is an urge to cling emotionally to the lost person as long as possible, and, on the other, the disengagement from him or her.

The process of psychological distancing is described by Freud (p. 154) in the following terms:

> The task is now carried through bit by bit, under great expense of time and cathectic energy, while all the time the existence of the lost object is continued in the mind. Each single one of the memories and hopes which bound the libido to the object is brought up and hyper-cathected, and the detachment of the libido from it accomplished. Why this process of carrying out the behest of reality bit by bit, which is in a nature of a compromise, should be so extraordinarily painful is not at all easy to explain in terms of mental economics.

In more personal terms, the work of mourning is described by one of Freud's followers, the psychoanalytic author and clinician Theodor Reik (Reik, 1940, p. 10 of Preface) ironically, in response to the loss of Freud himself to whom Reik was strongly attached:

> I know, now that the impression has passed, that we are called again to the labor of sorrow, that unseen, prolonged process of separation in which we take leave of our dear departed. It is work against great odds, for so many objects, places and circumstances remind us of the time he was still with us. How can we accomplish this work which takes place so heartbreakingly in the midst of memory? Yet this silent process of the psyche is necessary, for our energy must be dedicated to the demands of the day.

These are two complex statements which summarize a number of distinct insights about the nature of mourning. To begin with, we are dealing with the process in which the individual does not wish to take part, a struggle not of his own choosing with which he finds himself obliged to cope. No one mourns because they really want to. On the contrary, mourning is a process of compulsory adjustment.

Why resistance to mourning? Resistance stems from the very nature of affective attachments. According to Freud, affective attachments are build on a foundation of psychic energy—it takes energy to build them, and, conversely, it takes perhaps even more energy to take them apart. Emotional connections are, in a manner of speaking, stabilized energy. Because the psyche is essentially conservative which means not eager to change patterns of emotional investment, attachments are not dissolved automatically in response to a loss. They do not simply fade away. They are taken apart, at a psychological cost to the person.

Freud made an additional observation about the process of mourning. He remarked that the memories and hopes which bound us affectively to the lost person are revived, in fact, they return to the awareness with added emotional charge. This effectively means that, in order to forget, one must first remember vividly, i.e., one must experience, often in a forceful way, that which one is seeking to put behind psychologically. Thus, in order to mourn successfully, one must be willing to take a risk of experiencing something in an unwelcome way.

One might say that mourning is a form of emotional revival which has more to do with re-experiencing than with remembering. Clearly, this would imply a state of considerable emotional vulnerability. The vulnerability is exacerbated by the fact that the emotional revival of memories in mourning is not a predictable process. Neither the patient nor the therapist can anticipate which memories will be brought forth and with what emotional force.

Remembering in mourning is rarely a serene reminiscence; and it rarely unfolds in a smooth sequence. Rather, it can have a fitful, spasmodic course (more of a smooth muscle contraction than smooth sailing).

It is a process which is not really under the patient's conscious control; one does not start out with an agenda. Once begun, the emotional revival of memories can acquire a momentum of its own with fits and starts. The unpredictable nature of this process is something the patient senses—somehow—and fears. Therefore, he or she needs support from the therapist to ensure that mourning is not stopped prematurely, i.e. before a sense of relief and closure have been achieved.

Our discussion of mourning should be qualified by pointing out that not all people mourn with the same intensity and that a stormy course is not inevitable. The nature, as well as depth of attachment, vary from individual to individual, and so does the manner in which they respond to disruption and losses in their lives. However, in clinical settings, it is by no means uncommon to encounter the more intense forms of mourning described above. For that reason, it would be helpful if the therapist were able to recognize that the disruptive and unpredictable nature of the process of mourning is a part of a well-known pattern, as opposed to being an aberration from some ideal smooth way of coping with loss.

The process of mourning entails not only active working through of revived affect and memories, but also the opposing psychological force which drives the person to return to the business of living. This is a natural, self-protective mechanism to ensure that the person will be mobilized out of their grief, back into the external world to respond again to life's demands, opportunities and other people. Thus, the natural outcome of normal mourning is expected to be favorable, and the process itself self-limited.

Complicated mourning

In his work with patients who had suffered a loss, Freud observed that some forms of mourning were accompanied by a marked loss of self-esteem, whereas others were not. He maintained that the loss of self-esteem was absent in normal grief. However, in other, more complicated forms of mourning, the loss of self-esteem was particularly striking. It manifested itself in highly critical statements that patients made about themselves. These self-critical statements were not only very poignant and elaborate, but they appeared quite unrealistic.

After struggling to account for this paradoxical situation, Freud eventually concluded that the exaggerated self-criticism was in fact directed towards the person whom the patient had lost (through death or disappointment). It was a part of the emotional response towards another person. One is dealing then with an ambivalent attachment, that is to say one in which a strong attachment is complicated by hostile feelings which the patient cannot accept or deal with in some simple way.

Freud concluded from the self-hate he observed in patients with complicated mourning, that they acted as if the anger and hostility they felt toward the love object had now been absorbed (through a process called identification) into oneself and then turned against oneself.

This mechanism of internalizing experience permits the person who is grieving to hold onto the lost love object psychologically, if they cannot hold onto it in reality. It is a substitute for the lost "real thing" and its function is to ensure that "the existence of the lost object is continued in the mind" (Freud, 1917, p. 154). Thus, "in spite of the conflict with the loved person the love relation need not be given up." (p. 160).

This defensive mechanism is intended to spare the person the impact of loss. However, this relief comes at a psychological cost to the bereaved person, namely the internalized hostility is now turned against the self. It is easy to see how this process would lay foundation for the development of depressive states and depressive vulnerability is indeed one of the major consequences of identifications of this type.

Another feature of the process of identification is that it is unconscious—it is not someone's chosen conscious strategy for overcoming a loss. It is, in a sense, a protective settlement which has been negotiated out of awareness to save time and spare the person psychological pain. Thus, the advantage of unconscious defenses is that they operate automatically and protect without expending much energy which is typically required for thinking things through very carefully and considering only the best options.

The automatic nature of the defense mechanisms can be compared to the way in which spinal and cerebellar mechanisms adjust posture after someone trips. If we needed to reason through every postural adjustment, we could not really walk.

On the other hand, because these protective psychic mechanisms are not conscious, they are not easily detected or controlled, and they cannot be simply turned on and off at will. As important as they are in shielding the person from the full impact of an experience, they are only partial solutions.

The loss of someone who was ambivalently loved is not the only loss which can trigger complicated mourning. Freud noted that it could also occur in response to losing something more abstract with which the person is strongly involved emotionally, such as, for example, one's country, or liberty, or an ideal (Freud, 1917, p. 153).

This observation has important implications. It permits us to expand the definition of loss to include a variety of life's circumstances, particularly traumatic circumstances, because trauma and loss share a good deal of common ground emotionally. One can grieve for someone, but one can also grieve for loss of something.

It is advantageous to be able to identify as loss circumstances and events other than the loss of a loved one .The advantage lies in being able to identify important common features in a variety of psychological reactions and difficulties which seemingly have nothing in common. Also, once a loss has been identified, one is in a position to anticipate mourning. The reverse can also occur. If the patient's reactions are identified as mourning, one can begin to look for a loss that the patient may not be aware of or that has somehow been obscured.

Similarities between mourning and traumatic reactions

Clinicians who deal with post-traumatic states will note that the process of mourning, as described earlier, with its revival of affect and painful return of memories which bound the person to the lost love object resembles greatly reactions to trauma. In our view, post-traumatic reactions and mourning (especially complicated mourning) share two significant similarities. The first one is the often laborious course of the process of working through. We might refer to this feature as the spasmodic quality of grieving. The second similarity has to do with *internalizing* some aspect of the traumatic situation.

Character of the mourning process

Post-traumatic reactions are often recognizable by the emergence of intense dysphoric affect, by agitation and a constant going back and forth between living in the present and living in the past, and by what appears to others as obsessional preoccupation with the traumatic situation. The patient appears as if they were on a roller-coaster and had no choice about remembering and re-experiencing the past. When specific elements of the traumatic situation are remembered, they seem to be recalled with emotional force, as though the experience were ongoing or had just occurred.

This laborious integration of the traumatic experience, "bit by bit", as opposed to some smooth and modulated sequence, is also very characteristic of the course in which traumatic reactions resolve themselves. All of these features strongly resemble the nature of the mourning process.

The role of internalization

One of Freud's most important and influential contributions is his view that reactions to loss entail internalization of experience. Internalization is a process whereby some experience or emotional situation is absorbed into the psychic life of an individual. Once absorbed, it continues to exert an influence on how a person feels and acts. It is a trace or a residue of an experience, but an active trace which alters, as it were, the psychological landscape into which it has been absorbed. This process operates unconsciously and its impact cannot be readily detected.

In the case of complicated mourning, this process of internalization takes the form of identification with the lost love object. Identification is a mechanism which has the specific function of repairing the sense of rupture and a painful discontinuity which stem from loss. However, as is evident from the previous discussion, this benefit occurs at a cost. Namely, in internalizing the lost person through identification, one is also internalizing, i.e. absorbing psychologically the entire emotional climate of that relationship.

Freud focused specifically on ambivalent attachments, because there, the identification entails absorbing hostility which tends to be turned against the self, leading to depressive states. Thus, one cannot simply identify with the lost love object without placing oneself at risk for absorbing the painful affect as well. This means that identification as a means of overcoming the loss makes one's inner world a great deal more complex, often leading to dysphoria and perhaps depression as well. Even if no major depressive state ensues, the added psychological complexity leaves the person with something to resolve.

The internalized material is not a memory, or is certainly not just a memory. It is, in a sense, an emotional memory, an affective inheritance from a significant earlier situation which carries over into the present and has an impact on how a person feels or perceives things. From the psychodynamic point of view, the internalized material is a major player.

Internalization mechanisms operate in traumatic situations as well (abuse situations, wars etc.). However, instead of an identification with the lost love object, the person internalizes significant aspects of the traumatic situation, typically the relationship with the person who traumatized them in some way.

Internalization is common in situations in which a person is too vulnerable to oppose the aggressor and fight them effectively—for example, children in abuse situations, adults in abuse situations or war victims. Thus, if a realistic defense is not feasible for fear of retaliation, the relationship with the aggressor will be internalized. In this way, the aggressor can be opposed and fought internally.

Transferring the field of battle into one's inner world provides a measure of control when control cannot be achieved in any objective way, because the person being traumatized is too young or they have been weakened by circumstances. Providing a measure of control is a critical advantage of internalization in a traumatic situation. However unpleasant the ongoing emotional struggle with an internalized hostile relationship may prove to be, the fact that it takes place within the confines of one's own personality, as opposed to being turned on and off by the aggressor, affords a sense of control. The struggle is now felt to be contained psychologically—somehow—within one's inner world. While this can bring a good deal of pain—dysphoric states, anger, anxiety and other accompanying features—still, the struggle has been *localized*, from the patient's' point of view. This is important in and of itself.

There are two types of traumatic situations which are especially relevant clinically: psychological abuse or traumatization and sexual traumatization.

Psychological traumatization

Psychological traumatization can occur in a wide range of interpersonal circumstances, and for a variety of reasons. However, those circumstances in which there is a very marked power differential between people involved have a potential for being especially traumatogenic. Wars, employment settings and families, as different as they are, share the common element of difference in personal power. Some participants, by virtue of their role (legitimate or illegitimate), have a great deal of power, while others have very little. These three settings have, in turn, proven a frequent context for traumatization.

Family settings and traumatization

Traumatization of children by a parent is a paradigmatic case with obvious clinical significance. Complex as this subject is (and we shall not attempt to do it justice here), it shares with other traumatic situations an important psychological mechanism, namely, internalization. A father who is very harsh, punitive or stormy, impulsive, explosive or otherwise out of control, is likely to elicit fear and anger in the child. He may or may not be physically abusive as well.

Obviously, physical abuse would tend to greatly aggravate and complicate the picture. However, psychological traumatization can occur even without it, as a result of an ongoing fear, anticipation of danger, etc.

The relationship with the punitive father is internalized. The anger felt towards the father is a very important element of the internalized material. Once internalized, the anger is a problem for a number of different reasons. It is an unpleasant affective state, often accompanied by arousal or a sense of pressure which demands that the person articulate it somehow. Thus, anger creates a sense of inner imbalance.

If anger remains internalized, it may eventually turn into dysphoric and depressive states via the mechanism which we observed in mourning. In addition to having a potential for generating depression, anger towards the father is especially burdensome for the child because it readily generates guilt feelings. It is difficult to avoid guilt feelings because, alongside the resentment for ill-treatment, the child also feels love towards the father and has an ongoing need to be loved in turn, to be admired, approved of etc. He is highly dependent, both psychologically and in terms of daily support and resources. This dependence is not a brief or transient state, and the child has no choice about it.

The guilt feelings generated by anger towards the parent are a particularly troublesome aspect of traumatic reactions. They cannot be simply talked away. Traumatized individuals may be exquisitely aware of them, or they may be completely unaware of them. Freud emphasized this aspect of reaction to trauma in his essay on Dostoevsky—"Dostoevsky and Parricide"—in which he described psychodynamics of abusive situations. (Freud, 1928).

Freud pointed out that guilt feelings may find expression in different actions and feelings. For example, the need for punishment may develop, more or less permanent, which may prompt the person to seek out, unconsciously, situations in which he will fail or be actively hurt.

The need to assuage guilt through precipitating failure and loss in one's life can endure well past the original traumatic situation in childhood—thus affecting disastrously one's entire life's pattern. Clinicians who work with patients who grew up in chaotic and traumatogenic environments are familiar with this particular life-pattern whereby the person seems plagued by setbacks and misfortune—although they appear to have the ability to do better. From a diagnostic point of view, it is important to distinguish problems which are due to genuine limitations in personal effectiveness and a lack of resources, from those which are due to a masked need to assuage guilt through failure. This can prove to be a significant diagnostic challenge. Yet it is important to successfully accomplish that task, because unexamined guilt feelings which operate through masochistic actions can be very persistent, and even when brought to light and interpreted, may prove very resistant to change.

Freud also postulated that guilt generated by intense hostility towards a tyrannical father could be expressed psychosomatically in hysterical symptoms. The person punishes themselves for a death wish by an unconscious identification with the person whom they wish dead—thus, penalty is extracted for a wish which is intolerable to the person, while the identity of the wish itself is obscured.

This particular conceptualization of a hysterical symptom as a possible defense against powerful hostility which the person is deeply invested in suppressing is helpful in dealing with traumatized individuals since feelings of anger and guilt in response to trauma figure prominently in those cases. Because anger and the accompanying guilt are a common (although not ubiquitous) affective response to being traumatized, it is important that both the patient and the therapist are aware of their existence, preferably in their naturally occurring and not disguised state.

This psychodynamic mechanism, elaborated by Freud, is only one pathway whereby symptoms are generated. Nevertheless, it is of special relevance in trauma cases because it permits us to tie conceptually a number of distinct issues and difficulties whose joint occurrence in the patient's clinical picture is otherwise difficult to explain.

Instead of identifying with the hostile parent, the child may respond by internalizing only specific aspects of the parent. For example, if the father had been harsh and punitive, the child may have absorbed psychologically harshness and judgmental qualities which are then turned against him. This may eventually develop into very severe conscience (Freud, 1928).

While this particular consequence of being exposed to someone who was harsh and traumatizing is perhaps not quite as crippling psychologically as a compulsive need for atonement, it can nonetheless cause of a great deal of pain. It can lead to persistent states of acute self-doubt which can interfere with achievement, and can make it very difficult for the person to rejoice in and take credit for his or her achievement. Obviously, self-doubt can stem from any number of different sources. However, this mechanism is helpful to bear in mind when trying to conceptualize reactions to trauma, because it points out links among different elements of the clinical picture which are by no means self-evident. For example, when one is dealing with dysphoric and intropunitive patients it is not always evident at the outset whether this difficulty is a reflection of their depressive vulnerability or a result of an internalized traumatic relationship with a specific person.

Sexual traumatization

Sexual traumatization is another clinical domain of great complexity and importance. Its adverse effects are numerous, and its impact has been widely recognized and appreciated. It continues to be recognized as a powerful source of a whole range of different symptoms. Psychological symptoms, as well as some important dynamic issues associated with sexual traumatization were reviewed in Section I of this book—"Psychological Disturbances in Patients with Pseudoseizures". In this section, we shall focus on a particular psychodynamic mechanism which plays an important role in the pathogenesis. This mechanism accounts for some of the complexity and perhaps unique difficulties which reactions to sexual traumatization can involve.

Sandor Ferenczi (1873–1933), one of the most prominent of psychoanalytic clinicians and a colleague of Freud, dealt very intensively with the issues involved in sexual traumatization and its long-term consequences for the affective and personality development of children. He made several important observations about the internalization mechanisms which are evoked in that situation (Ferenczi, 1949): "The weak and undeveloped personality reacts to sudden unpleasure, not by defense but by an anxiety—ridden identification and by introjection of the menacing person or aggressor." (p. 228).

As the above description indicates, identification with the aggressor occurs as a part of the reaction to sexual trauma. As will be recalled from the earlier discussion, this mechanism is shared with other forms of traumatization and for much the same reasons—the vulnerability of the victim, in this case, because of his or her youth.

Ferenczi goes on to elaborate the process of identification: "Through the identification, or let us say, the introjection of the aggressor, he disappears as part of the external reality, and becomes intra- instead of extra-psychic" (p. 228).

Ferenczi made an important observation concerning the next step in the process of the identification. He pointed out that that which had been internalized could subsequently be modified or changed in the sense that external events or people could not. Thus, the full adverse impact of the traumatic experience can be lessened. "In any case the attack as rigid external reality ceases to exist" (p. 228).

In this respect as well, the internalization process in response to sexual trauma shares common ground with internalization mechanisms in other forms of traumatic experience.

Ferenczi pointed out an additional aspect of the identification process which is specifically relevant to sexual traumatization:

> The most important change, produced in the mind of the child by the anxiety- ridden identification with the adult partner, is the introjection of the guilt feelings of the adult which makes hitherto harmless play appear as a punishable offence (p. 228).

This is a particularly burdensome aspect of internalization in sexual trauma, namely that the guilt feelings are internalized as part of the identification, although they cannot be linked rationally in any way to the child. They literally belong to the other person. Yet the victim is blamed anyway, and she (or he) eventually blames herself over an action in which she participated on terms which are not blameworthy. The terms of adult sexuality are superimposed on an earlier event which, from the child's point of view, may have had a different meaning, or may not have had any meaning at all. Guilt or shame (the latter is probably an even more influential factor) are thus inherited as a part of the unconscious process which is otherwise aimed at providing relief and defense. They are not a part of the original meaning of the experience, rather, they are feelings in which the victim subsequently finds herself trapped.

Because guilt and shame do not stem from a consciously decided upon action, but are something which is inherited as a painful by-product of a defense strategy, their presence is seen as something outrageous, yet difficult to eliminate. The patient may feel, in rapid succession, both shame and anger at being ashamed, since it certainly makes no sense for the victim to be ashamed. This is an experience which is very self-alienating and involves feeling, often in a very acute and bizarre way, gaps emerging in one's sense of self. It is a direct threat to the sense of the continuity of self. It can fuel affective storms or even lead, in some fragile patients, to states of acute confusion and dissociation.

The role of internalization and dissociation in pseudoseizures

- Identification with traumatized parent
- Anger dynamics
  - When is an accident an accident?
  - Anger turned against the self vs anger projected
- The role of dissociation
- Dynamic functions of pseudoseizures

Identification with the traumatized parent and the masochistic lifestyle

The preceding discussion dealt with the process of internalization which is an important part of the response to trauma. Internalization is not a single mechanism, rather, it can lead to very diverse defensive scenarios.

Identification is an important mechanism of internalization which will be reviewed here in some detail, because it plays a significant part in the dynamics of post-traumatic response. As will be recalled from our earlier discussion, identification with the parent or an introjection of the parental image has to do with internalizing the parent as a whole, or, in some cases, a particular aspect of the relationship to him or her.

The process of identification is especially pertinent in a subgroup of female patients with pseudoseizures. This is a group of patients who grew up in traumatic, difficult or chaotic backgrounds and whose mothers were either victims of traumatization, or may have had a more generally difficult life course. The mothers were victims, or were experienced as such by their daughters.

An identification with the mother who was traumatized in some significant way is a powerful source of difficulty as it often results in an unconscious adoption of a victim life-style. This life-style consists of a whole range of painful circumstances. Especially noteworthy is a pervasive lack of initiative and assertiveness in pursuit of one's legitimate goals. In this context, the victim life-style is not due to a lack of ability. On the contrary, there is often the impression that there is a potential to do better, yet there is a continuing discrepancy between what the person is able to do (or appears able to do) and their consistently troubled lives.

Identification is not a conscious decision to relive someone's troubled life. It is an unconscious process which the person in no way intended. They are not choosing to behave in self-defeating ways. The process of identification is very insidious and one can only reconstruct it from evidence which has accumulated along the way—i.e., from a variety of bad outcomes in the patient's life. Identification with a mother who was a victim in some way impairs initiative and the readiness to use one's energy and ability in pursuit of one's own life. Thus, the identification of this kind blocks access to one's own resources. The patient behaves *as if* she identified with the traumatized parent.

This concept appears very counterintuitive, because we are used to defense mechanisms which are primarily oriented toward relieving pain and not augmenting it.

Freud discovered that the process of identification occurred as a response to a traumatic loss. It is a part of the grieving process, a way of not giving up the lost person completely. It is easier to accept that the identification with the mother would occur as a specific part of grieving for a mother who died prematurely or traumatically .The identification in this context functions as a response to traumatic loss. On the other hand, the identification with a mother who has lead a difficult life is much less straightforward. This is not an acute event and it involves no apparent grieving.

Overt grieving in acute stages makes a good deal of sense to both the patient and the clinician. It seems very normal and very appropriate. While people very in the extent to which they are willing to engage in expressions of grieving, and they sometimes claim to be ashamed of it, they are rarely truly ashamed of grieving in response to an obvious loss.

Grieving has a very definite target. The loss of a parent is an event with a very clear traumatic focus (a high-definition event in psychological terms). However, when dealing with an identification with a parent who had a difficult life, one is not confronting a well-defined loss.

It may not be immediately apparent whether, in a particular woman's life, an identification with the traumatized parent played a destructive role, and what psychological ends this served, until one has understood the psychodynamics of that particular case a great deal better. This process typically requires a good deal of time and reconstructive effort.

It may be helpful to conceptualize identification with the traumatized mother as an accumulation of many small instances of grieving. This may not be accompanied by overt sadness, but it is like grieving in that the patient does not approach the business of living with the force and energy which might be expected given her abilities. The patient behaves *as if* she were chronically grieving.

Identification with a traumatized parent is like grieving—not for a single—but for a *whole series of insidious and poorly defined losses*. If the mother has lead a generally difficult and traumatic life, the patient, and the therapist trying to help them, are obliged to confront a number of losses some of which may be poorly defined and poorly remembered. A poorly defined and poorly remembered loss is a significant therapeutic challenge (it does not look like a loss, but it *behaves* like a loss).

A question arises as to why we should attempt to understand the workings of this elusive mechanism. Understanding this dynamic mechanism is important, because identification with the traumatized parent does a great deal more than just affect unfavorably the outcome of a single event in the daughter's life. Rather, its impact is evident in many domains of a person's life. It insidiously shapes the entire approach to life. It organizes behavior toward hardship and defeat rather than success.

It is not just a question of making the daughter more vulnerable to depression, or some other specific symptomatology although this can certainly occur. Identification does more than just increase the likelihood of specific conflicts. It has an impact which is pervasive yet hard to trace to any specific event or cause.

In discussing this particular psychodynamic mechanism, it should be pointed out that the identification with the parent of the same gender is not a pathogenic process per se. It is not there in order to generate pathology. Quite the opposite, it is a major mechanism of psychosocial development which supports development of the appropriate gender identity. Without being able to identify with their mothers, female children could not acquire a model of feminine identity.

Acquisition of gender identity is a complex process which is not limited to a few skills. On the contrary, it involves a wide range of attitudes, aptitudes and behaviors. This process would be far too long and laborious if each skill and behavior had to be explicitly outlined and painstakingly acquired.

The identification with a traumatized parent, especially the mother, or, more precisely, *internalization of the traumatic background of the mother's life,* is a significant source of difficulty which shapes the clinical picture in a significant proportion of women patients with such background. We cannot determine with certainty what proportion of female children with such backgrounds internalize the traumatic background of the parent with serious adverse consequences, so that it becomes a significant psychological burden and blocks their initiative and their pursuit of constructive goals. Obviously, not everyone faced with traumatized parents evolves psychologically in such a direction. Indeed, when faced with traumatic events of any kind, people vary greatly in their resilience and adaptability, as well as their choice of methods in confronting the problem.

Nonetheless, in dealing with post-traumatic pseudoseizure patients, especially women patients, we found that the internalization of the traumatic background of the mother's life played a powerful, albeit an insidious role in a significant subset of cases. It does not play such a role in all pseudoseizure patients. In other patients, other mechanisms are more prominent and determine the clinical picture.

The idea that the patient's persisting difficulties might be due to the identification with the traumatized mother is not a notion which typically occurs at the outset of therapy. It is much more common to begin to consider this possibility after the patient has presented a good deal of material which reveals a whole series of trouble points in her life. Some of them are acute and some are ongoing, some never get resolved and some do. What is characteristic is that the overall level and presence of difficulty remain constant (the baseline does not change). It has to be pointed out that the patient may remain very active and engaged in trying to cope with the difficulties, yet the overall background of a troubled life does not substantially change in spite of this effort.

Reviewing a patient's life in therapy and finding that it has this persistently troubled quality ("crisis normal", as one patient put it) is not unusual. After all, patients usually come to therapy in order to review their difficulties and find some form of relief and resolution. Furthermore, the patients who have been traumatized themselves often present with histories which are rich in symptoms and difficulties. Patients who are poor are especially vulnerable to being traumatized. An important task for the therapist is to establish to what extent the patient's difficulties reflect specifically the identification with the traumatized mother.

While it is very true that the different factors mentioned above may generate similar clinical presentations, the clinical picture and implications for outcome are not the same in each case. Internalization of the traumatic background of the mother's life can have a pervasive adverse influence. Not only can it represent a significant burden in coping with life—it creates an attitude whereby a series of disasters are accepted as one's lot. They are experienced emotionally as being nothing unusual.

This is not a conscious attitude, nor does the patient have a clearly formulated masochistic plan for their life. The patient would be quite surprised if someone asked her whether she believed that she was not entitled to any good fortune, nor to material security, nor to security in personal attachments.

No one would claim outright that these are merely dreams which are clearly beyond their reach and which are intended only for other people. Yet their life unfolds as though they believed it.

Individuals whose life brings many challenges question fate and the fairness of life. They can be outraged. A large number of them confront their difficulties, and some triumph over them. Accepting adversity as a matter of course, in fact, as one's due, is a signal that an identification with a traumatized or traumatically lost parent may have taken place. It is true that there are many individuals who are passive, and many who are depressed, as well as many who avoid facing life even in the absence of trauma. However, nothing is lost by bearing the possibility of identification in mind and exploring it with the patient.

Identification with the traumatized parent is more than an unpleasant aspect of the clinical picture. It is an active obstacle to the patient's accomplishing his or her life. In those patients who have also been traumatized themselves, it presents a major obstacle in mobilizing those resources which they do have to fight the trauma and reduce its impact (analogous to having a frozen bank account after one's house has been robbed). It is an added burden in an already challenging situation. For this reason, the threshold for exploring this topic should be fairly low. Nothing is lost if we discover that this problem does not exist—in fact, the absence of adverse identification is an asset in mobilizing a person's resources just as it is reassuring for the coach to know that the runner has no allergies.

The issue of survivor guilt

When dealing with the issue of identification with a traumatized parent, a question arises as to why this particular mechanism is activated, or why some women absorb the traumatic background of their mother's lives.

Living in a setting where one witnesses daily some ongoing difficulty or controversy or struggle is a source of chronic emotional tension. This is especially true if the mother is struggling, or is not treated well and the child is powerless to stop it. This tension is built from an intolerable cognitive dissonance—the sharp discrepancy between how things should be and how they are. Being acutely aware of one's powerlessness to change a bad situation which one very much wants to change and which is affecting someone one cares about is very painful. Repeatedly experiencing such a sense of powerlessness means to be continuously conflicted. Such a state is very destructive to one's sense of self-esteem and self-efficacy. A particular burden of this situation is that it often generates powerful guilt feelings.

One might argue that a child is certainly in no position to change things, and cannot be expected to do so. Consequently, any guilt feelings stemming from his inability to "rescue" his/her mother from the painful circumstances of her life are quite irrational. While such feelings are clearly irrational, they are nonetheless also very real and very common.

The child feels as though she (or he) abandoned the mother to her fate, and since the mother's history cannot be changed retroactively, the only way to put it right is to feel the way she felt—i.e., immobilized. The child thus takes on the burden of the mother's affect. In a sense, the child is making an unconscious attempt at reparation "I could not, and did not prevent her from experiencing bad things, so, in order to make up for it, I will feel what she felt." The guilt feelings are diminished in the process of taking on someone's depressed affect or their sense of immobilization.

Not only the guilt feelings, but also the sense of intense resentment and anguish which accompanies witnessing situations which one is powerless to change diminish through identification. Thus, the affective burden of that situation is lessened markedly. It is true that another kind of burden is taken on, namely the sense of failure and depressiveness, but this burden is considered less intolerable and is less threatening than the feelings of intense guilt and acute conflict.

The identification in this particular situation functions as a powerful (albeit costly) defense against feelings which are especially intolerable and which cannot be handled otherwise. It is not a simple defense. Rather, it is a way of stabilizing and reorganizing a good deal of emotional experience and emotional history.

This defense is especially likely to arise in a situation in which a person is powerless, either by virtue of being a child, or is facing circumstances of special adversity, such as war. The presence of a support system of any kind, or resources which the individual can use—that is, assets of any type which reduce a person's sense of powerlessness—all function as a powerful shield which reduces the likelihood of harmful introjections.

As we have noted earlier, the process of internalizing the traumatic background of the parent's life is not apparent when it is going on. Its impact may not become apparent until much later. The consequences need not be dramatic, and they need not entail a whole series of failures or disasters. The impact could be felt indirectly, for example, as fear of success. The daughter feels reluctant to fulfill all her potential for success and may unconsciously fear rather than pursue material and emotional security, because this is experienced as the betrayal of the mother, a form of disloyalty to her, even an act of aggression towards her.

Such a point of view is of course not consciously held by the daughter. It is so completely and obviously irrational and unreasonable that it cannot long survive as a conscious thought which is subject to ongoing critical logical appraisal.

However, this point of view is not a delusional idea, but an unconscious motivation. As a result of this compelling but poorly understood motivation, the person labors under the affective burden of feeling guilty unless he or she fails. This affective burden is perhaps even more difficult to confront directly than irrational thoughts would be.

Points of technique

Motivation to fail which is engendered by guilt feelings is far from easy to accept from the patient's point of view and is not easy for the therapist either. It is important that the idea be introduced to the patient with considerable care. It is especially important that the patient in no way feels as though they were being told that they were their own worst enemy. While their lives may be unfolding in an unfavorable direction, this is not because they wish to be their own worst enemy, but because they are burdened by unconscious motivation. This motivation, in turn, stems from an identification which occurred to provide relief from intense conflict, helplessness and guilt feelings—feelings which occurred at the time when the child did not, in fact, have any ready means of changing the situation. People do not choose their defense mechanism from a menu.

Defensive identification with the traumatized parent is a very legitimate reason for what appears to outsiders as a self-defeating life course. It in no way implies that the person is their own worst enemy. It does imply that they are defending themselves from a poorly understood threat and the need to defend against that threat takes precedence over other—more reasonable goals.

With this understanding in mind, one is able to approach the patient, not as someone who is "their own worst enemy", but as someone who had, in a sense, made the best of a bad situation. The patient is seen not so much as someone who is masochistic, but as someone who had made a bad bargain in emotional terms, a bad bargain based on a desire to make reparation. This bargain needs to be reevaluated to determine if other and better options are now possible

One possible way of introducing the topic would be to ask the patient, "*In addition to* feeling bad for your mother, would it be OK to also *enjoy* life, or have fun, or do something which would bring you reward? *Is it* OK to have good things happen too? What is OK and what is too much?"

These questions may sound very odd, but they really reflect what the patient actually feels at some level without recognizing it.

The above statements are introducing the idea to the patient that they are, in fact, making a decision about how much good they are allowing into their lives (as odd as that may seem), that they are, in fact, restricting themselves, introducing limits.

The idea that one could be threatened by the possibility of a successful and prosperous life is very counterintuitive. It goes against all our usual ideas about our goals and our lives. It does not have any obvious and clear explanation for being there. Consequently, this notion could be very threatening to the patient.

To reduce the potential threat to the patient, the therapist may attempt to deal with the masochistic or self-defeating elements of the identification as a form of mourning. Reconceptualizing seemingly masochistic phenomena as a form of mourning removes the threat for the patient of "being their own worst enemy". Mourning is not in any way self-defeating or odd or embarrassing. It is consistent with the feelings which are already very much in evidence in the patient's life: immobilization, the fear of initiative, mild depressiveness. To mourn someone is very different from a defensive identification with a masochistic outcome.

One might suggest this to the patient in the following way: *"You are acting as if you had lost something, or lost something which is very necessary to face life. You act as if you were grieving."*

The phrase *as if* is important here, because it helps to qualify what can otherwise be too strong a statement. The therapist is not stating boldly that the patient is mourning when no overt signs of grieving are in evidence. The statement is an attempt to provide the patient with a new angle or a new framework for some of her troublesome affects.

Reconceptualizing defensive identification with a traumatized parent as a form of chronic grieving is therapeutic for yet another reason. To grieve is a conscious act. It is a volitional act, albeit an unpleasant one. While grieving may be intense and unwelcome, the person who grieves is still somewhat in control. Identification, however, is based on an unconscious motivation which shapes one's actions in an insidious way. To be at the mercy of such a process can only make one feel powerless in circumstances in which one no longer has a reason to feel powerless.

Reconceptualizing identification as mourning frees one to experience certain specific affects instead of a poorly characterized and chronic sense of ineffectivenss. For example, a person can feel sad for her mother, or angry at her fate, or angry with her, instead of feeling exactly what the mother felt. Anger, grief and compassion are specific affects, not a diffuse affective blend. It is easier—in the long run—to deal with particular affects than with vague blends. Particular affects have specific names, they can usually be attached to specific situations, people and circumstances, and they can be placed in time. It is easier to control well-characterized affects than vague negative affect for which it is difficult to say when it began and who is involved and why. To mourn for someone, or be angry at what happened to them, or to be angry with them, is not the same as taking on their life's path as one's own. In fact, mourning may prevent such an outcome.

It should be pointed out that deconstructing the identification with a traumatized parent is a process, and not a single event. It cannot be accomplished as a result of a single therapeutic intervention. In deconstructing an identification one is actually *changing the internal organization of particular affect and experience*. This process is somewhat *like pulling strands from a cloth* or even removing one of the beams from the roof of the house. This could be quite uncomfortable for the patient and it is not unusual to encounter anger and resistance. A new structure or organization needs to be built gradually to replace what had to be changed. Fully understanding that this process requires time is important. Thus, neither the patient nor the therapist should feel that they are failing if they cannot resolve this issue smoothly and rapidly.

In addition to reconceptualizing identification as mourning, there is another therapeutic goal to be achieved here, namely dealing with the maternal image as being fully that of a victim. Imagining or remembering the mother as solely a victim creates a sense of helplessness. One cannot simply dispel this image or change it abruptly. However, while allowing that the mother indeed led a difficult life, and acknowledging that the patient is right to feel badly for her, one can also encourage the patient to seek for evidence of strength and effectiveness in her mother. Eventually, a modified image of the mother can emerge: she was somewhat of a victim, but also somewhat of a success. This image does not deny her traumatic life, and does not completely negate the daughter's experience of her as a victim, but it also allows for a strong and effective side. Not feeling compelled to see her in extreme terms is a form of significant emotional growth.

Recognizing the mother's strength and effectiveness, in turn, makes it possible for the daughter to accept her own strength and power without being threatened by them, or worse, experiencing them as an act of betrayal of the mother.

This particular emotional link between one's own success and betrayal of the traumatized parent to whom one continues to be attached is probably one of the most destructive psychodynamic patterns. Its impact can probably match and sometimes exceed many an overt traumatic event. As paradoxical as it may seem, abusers and aggressors who come and go are perhaps easier to deal with because the victim, of necessity, has to mobilize and mobilize against them. Identification with an attachment figure who was traumatized is a completely opposite process. It represents an attempt—and an unconscious one at that—to maintain another person psychologically when they could not be rescued in reality. It amounts to a debilitating way of loving. Yet the person whose experience is organized in this way does not feel that there is anything wrong. Thus, it is a burden against which the person cannot get easily mobilized.

It should be noted that the impact of an identification with a traumatized parent can vary considerably. Consequently, the degree of therapeutic effort which needs to be mobilized in order to deal with this challenge can also vary. One of the important components of that effort includes reconceptualizing the mother as someone who was not quite the same person as the daughter's retained image of her. Eventually, she will be understood to be, in emotional terms, someone who *is not fully contained within this unvarying memory*.

As a consequence of this effort, being strong and effective would no longer be experienced as something the patient's mother did not do, but rather as something she was not recognized for at that time. Allowing for maternal strength and effectiveness to emerge frees the daughter from a rigid (albeit unconscious) loyalty to the maternal immobilization since that immobilization has now been challenged as a pervasive reality.

In the course of this therapeutic intervention, the patient is thus not asked to completely undo the identification with her mother which is impossible anyway, but to identify with a more complete and perhaps more balanced image of her.

The superwoman challenge

Internalizing the traumatic background of a parent's life is not the only way of coming to terms with this challenge. Not infrequently, individuals who were forced to remain aware of the traumatic background of the parent's life emerge highly motivated to become strong and effective. This motivation is often manifested in a strong need to take charge of difficult situations, and not allow them to deteriorate (orientation towards prevention of disasters). A certain proportion of pseudoseizure patients fall into this category.

The life's path of individuals in this category evolves through their intense efforts to avoid repeating their mother's life at all costs. This motivation can and often does lead to individuals who possess considerable competence and merit.

While this path is obviously preferable to the internalization of the traumatic background of the parent's life, it is not without problems of its own. The problems are related to the fact that this particular motivation is largely based on fear. It confines the person to recognizing only two extreme ways of being: a superwoman, or if not a superwoman, then necessarily a victim. The person operates under an ongoing burden which causes them to feel that, if they relax their efforts, they will necessarily and inevitably regress to a position of humiliating passivity and failure. Thus, they see themselves as always potentially in danger of failing, even when they are strong.

Pseudoseizure patients with a superwoman orientation show a strong tendency to devote nearly all of their organizational ability and competence into taking care of numerous difficulties and family responsibilities. Rarely rewarded, they are always working. Often they find themselves surrounded by circumstances and individuals replete with problems of all kinds which they are obliged to manage. Their energy is thus largely absorbed in the process of evading disasters or managing them for other people. Theirs is a perpetual stance of an unpaid and unrecognized nurse and unpaid and unrecognized counselor. This implies that very little energy remains which can be used to chart an independent path of personal development towards educational and professional goals. They seem reluctant to deliberately invest into something which benefits them obviously or directly.

Involvement with the difficulties of others is not a problem per se. It becomes a problem when such involvement is continuous and excessive, and does not allow for any time or resources to be used in the pursuit of those educational and professional goals which the person's abilities would normally entitle them to pursue.

The second difficulty has to do with the person's involvement being significantly motivated by an unconscious need to seek out troubled circumstances or people in order to give herself the opportunity to experience a sense of mastery. Paradoxically, a permanent sense of mastery is rarely achieved.

Unconscious motivation of this kind is painful. It is compulsive, rather than volitional. It tends to organize behavior around circumstances which are more complex and difficult than they need to be, and which the person would not choose if they were not working psychologically to counteract the impact of the parent's traumatic background.

Finding a balance between needs which stem from our involvement with others and needs which have to do with personal growth and security is not a simple task even in nonclinical settings. One need not have psychological problems to find it challenging. However, if the person's motivation is derived chiefly from the need to overcompensate in order to defend herself against the danger of reliving the traumatic background of her mother's life, then the person may have any number of achievements but no feelings of success.

The concept of defensive identification with a traumatized parent enables us to understand that people can be *substantially hurt psychologically even when they themselves were not traumatized*. It is a source of difficulty in and of itself. This is far from being an esoteric theoretical issue. Quite the contrary, it is an issue of great practical significance for any therapist who is trying to mobilize patients, including pseudoseizure patients, who are stuck in unfavorable circumstances. For patients who were themselves traumatized, this identification represents a liability which drains their motivation to get better. It is a stubborn albeit often unrecognized obstacle.

In our discussion of the impact of this important dynamics we focused on women patients. It should be pointed out, however, that an identification with a traumatized parent is by no means limited to women. Men are just as affected by an empathic identification with a traumatized parent. It has a great psychodynamic significance for them as well (for example, it plays a role in the genesis of altruistic motivation and life-style). However, these psychodynamic ramifications will not be pursued in this context.

We should qualify our discussion by bearing in mind that, however compelling an internalization of the traumatic background of the parent's life might prove to be, it is by no means inevitable.

A mother who had had to face a lot of adversity can be experienced and remembered psychologically by the child as either a victim or a fighter. While we of course do not know what proportion of population belong to each category, it remains beyond doubt that both categories exist and that some women not only remember their mothers as "fighters", but perceive that role as their proud inheritance.

Perceiving one's mother as a fighter is psychologically empowering (she was a fighter and so am I). Perceiving her as a victim is psychologically debilitating (she was a victim and so am I). In helping our patients in the latter category we are acknowledging that their experience or perception of the mother as a victim might be real, but not unvarying. "Real, but not unvarying" means that other feelings and visions of the parent are possible and can be admitted into our experience and our emotional history and memory.

Anger dynamics

In addition to identification, there is another major challenge to dealing with traumatic circumstances. This challenge refers to the management of anger which arises in response to trauma. Anger is a natural and understandable response to trauma. It is not dysfunctional or pathological in and of itself.

There are forms of anger which stem from an empathic identification with those who have suffered. These forms of anger are a foundation of altruistic feelings and actions and they are indispensable.

In this discussion, however, we shall focus on forms of anger which are a source of concern for clinicians. A point of view has become established according to which anger is a sign that a person is out of control, that they are not in charge of the circumstances of their life, that their response is inadequate and blameworthy. In this view, anger serves as a final common pathway of failed adaptation.

There are situations in which all this might be true—a person is angry, because they cannot create a better response, because they are helpless or out of control. There are forms of anger and ways of expressing anger which are both frightening and blameworthy.

Ideas about anger as a consequence of failure in coping should come as conclusions at the end of an investigation of the patient's particular response, and not at the beginning. It matters whether anger is viewed as an end point and a failure, or as a part of the patient's overall history and dynamics.

If the view of anger as a failure of coping is a prelude to further exploration with a goal of understanding the patient better and helping him acquire better and more adaptive ways of approaching life, then this view can be constructive. If, however, it is a way of dismissing the patient, or assuming that his anger tells us all we need to know about him, then it is not constructive.

We are arguing for the position that anger is a common and natural response to trauma. It is very evident that people vary profoundly in the extent to which they manifest anger overtly. However, overt manifestations of anger are not a reliable guide to the actual importance of anger in the clinical picture of a given patient. Thus, the absence of manifest anger should not prevent us from trying to explore the possible role of anger in the person's response to trauma. By exploring, I mean to bear in mind the possibility that anger might be a part of the clinical picture.

A clinical situation in which anger is especially likely to play a role involves victims of motor vehicle accidents. I have explored important aspects of the dynamics of anger in the discussion of postconcussive/post-traumatic syndrome in Section I of this book ("Psychological Disturbances in Patients with Pseudoseizures"). In this context, I will discuss some additional features.

When is an accident an accident?

No one would question that genuine accidents can and do occur. Usually, we accept the view that an accident is something which was not intended. Some motor vehicle accidents do indeed occur by chance, and could not be considered anyone's fault. Others, however, while still called accidents, are clearly due to someone's error of judgment or poor driving skills. The latter category is large. Quite a few patients who developed the postconcussive/post-traumatic syndrome were victims of errors by other drivers. The fact that the accident was not intended does not mean that it was no one's fault. If it was indeed someone's fault, it is very likely that it will be processed psychologically as trauma, and not as an accident.

Motor vehicle collisions have a great potential to evoke a feeling of being in mortal danger. One need not necessarily be in a very dramatic accident to still become intensely frightened.

Consequences of the so-called mild head injury can be very persistent and very disruptive. The feelings of intense threat and subsequent hardships are not consistent with a psychological experience of an accident, but are highly consistent with an experience of *assault*. We cannot claim with certitude that all victims of motor vehicle accidents process them psychologically in this way, but a substantial proportion do, especially those who are struggling, and are very symptomatic and distressed. The fact that the person who caused the accident did not intend it does not mean that the victim will not process the experience as an assault.

Experiencing such an accident as an assault is not a conscious decision, nor is it due to a cognitive distortion. The patient with such an experience is not paranoid or delusional. Nor does he or she wish to have such an experience. We do not really know why people experience such accidents as an assault. This, however, should not prevent us from recognizing that they frequently do. We should recognize it, because if the patient experiences something as an assault, while others see it as an accident, a tension will arise which the patient will be obliged to deal with. He/she will likely experience the person who caused the accident as an aggressor, yet he will not be supported in this view by society at large, unless he or she brings a formal lawsuit and wins (which very few victims have resources to do).

A person who is a victim of mugging is recognized by society as a victim, and the person who assaulted them is an aggressor. The role of a victim of a motor vehicle accident is far more ambiguous. The patient who experiences the accident as an assault is likely to feel both angry and ashamed of feeling angry. They are trapped in feelings which they did not intend and which others do not validate.

Sensitivity to this particular dynamics is important, because it can help to reduce some of the intensity of the anger, as well as the patient's sense of isolation.

It should be added in this context that an accident can be processed as trauma even when it was not anyone's fault, or if no one else was involved, for example, a person ran into a tree. The experience of threat remains, the sense of confronting something which could harm us greatly. This is especially true of accidents which take place in work settings, for example, if a person loses an arm, because it got caught into a machine. This may have been no one's fault, but the experience of being assaulted is very likely to arise.

The psyche has great difficulty dealing with abstract dangers, because the possibility of something terrible occurring for no reason is too threatening. Under such circumstances, the aggressor is the fate or an inanimate object. We should point out that this is not a conscious viewpoint as much as it is an experience—the person experiences the machine, or fate, or a tree, *as if* they were an aggressor. In doing so, they are not consciously attributing human characteristics to nature or to machines. Rather, they are defensively adapting in order to avoid the even more threatening experience of living in a world which is random.

Anger turned against the self versus anger projected

Feelings of anger which are evoked in response to traumatic events present a challenge. The post-traumatic adaptation would be considerably simpler and shorter if anger could be dealt with (or disposed of) by a single psychological method and the resolution completed in a single moment. There are favorable circumstances in which this fast and effective resolution does indeed occur.

In clinical settings, however, one is much more likely to encounter individuals struggling with feelings of anger for protracted periods of time, relying on different methods with varying degrees of success.

Among the various methods employed one particular pattern occurs with some frequency. This pattern consists of two components which alternate with some regularity. The first component is characterized by internalizing the experience of anger (introjecting it). As a consequence of this, the person typically feels depressed, agitated and suffers from poor self-esteem (containment without resolution). In this phase of the process, anger is turned against the self.

When the person can no longer tolerate the negative affects associated with turning the anger against themselves, the second phase takes place in which the person operates under pressure to direct the anger away from oneself. The anger is projected outward. While this relieves some of the pressure which stems from the accumulated depressive affects and self-esteem problems, it generates another set of problems, namely, other people are now seen in a hostile light, and the world is experienced as threatening or impoverished. The predominant affective tone in this phase is phobic.

Thus, the person alternates between affective states in which anger is directed against himself/herself and those states in which it is projected onto others. His affective climate alternates between two equally painful extremes: I am bad or the world is bad. These are not conscious choices and the person is not paranoid. Rather, the unresolved anger which is dealt with in this particular way tends to generate an affective climate which is permeated by negative affects and a sense of insecurity.

The alternating or cyclical nature of these two phases (as opposed to each phase individually) is a clue that some unresolved traumatic material may be present. Usually, we tend to think of individuals as responding to anger primarily by one method, as opposed to the other. We do not expect to see intense shifts from one method to the other. A clinical picture which presents sharp contrasts and inconsistencies (a roller-coaster pattern) suggests that an unresolved traumatic focus might be present in which anger plays an important role.

Being caught in a bind between absorbing anger and projecting it is painful, especially if this process continues over extended periods of time, which it often does. Turning the anger against oneself and, alternatively, projecting it, are ways of containing anger without really dealing with it. They represent containment without resolution. They are not conscious strategies or plans for responding to anger, but are a part of a defensive mechanism which is triggered automatically to protect the person. This mechanism operates mostly unconsciously. It is something a person falls into or lapses into, rather than decides upon.

What does this particular defensive pattern of containing anger without really dealing with it accomplish for the person involved? It is helpful in a situation in which a person is passive or perceives himself/herself to be passive (response to sexual assault or sudden death of a loved one; war victims). Someone may feels helpless, because they lack the resources (especially true of children), or they fear that an assertive response would provoke retaliation.

Diffusing anger into depressive, phobic and agitated affects serves another very important function. It protects the individual from losing control over anger and acting out in a hostile way. The fear of loss of control and of acting out can pose an even greater emotional threat than the depressiveness and phobic quality of the environment. In a sense, the person buys the protection against the possibility of loss of control over anger at the cost of feeling unhappy and helpless.

It should be added that the fear of loss of control may not be fully realistic. The person may, if faced with anger explicitly, be able to respond appropriately. However, the defense is triggered to provide protection against something which is felt to be very dangerous at some fundamental and not easily accessible level. Thus, the sense of passivity and helplessness need not necessarily stem from the person's actual lack of resources.

A preoccupation with themes of power and powerlessness is another clue to unresolved anger (traumatically based). It should be pointed out that themes of power and helplessness are universal, and occur in the absence of traumatic events, merely as a response to daily life in society. However, an intense preoccupation with, or a persisting experience of, powerlessness points to unresolved, traumatically based anger.

The role of dissociation

Dissociation is a radical defensive strategy which is employed to protect the individual against traumatic danger of such magnitude or intensity that ordinary defensive operations are clearly inadequate to cope with it. It is a drastic intervention which is mobilized to prevent collapse.

Dissociation mechanisms have a place, both in the acute response to trauma, as well as in chronic adaptation to trauma. Dissociative episodes vary both in scope and complexity.

On an acute level, dissociation provides relief against intolerable dangers in someone's immediate environment (sexual assault, soldiers in battle, endangered civilians, as well as other traumatic events). It is a psychological and biological shield against terror.

Dissociation can also be incorporated into the person's ongoing post-traumatic adaptation. Here, it operates periodically, or recurrently. Recurrent episodes of dissociation can have the following functions. They shield the person against re-experiencing trauma in such as way as to be flooded by it. Dissociation is a barrier against the overwhelming intrusion of traumatic memory and its disorganizing affects. In addition, dissociation can serve as a defense against eruption of anger which is felt as a consequence of being traumatized.

Dissociation plays an important role in the psychodynamics of pseudoseizure syndromes. Pseudoseizures represent dissociative episodes in which the quality of consciousness changes markedly and the person is partly in contact with the present reality, and partly regressed which means that they are responding to the material from the past as if it were happening now. The material which emerges in such episodes is not clearly articulated. Often, only rudimentary phrases are uttered, usually reflecting traumatic content, in the setting of confusion and agitation.

During these episodes, the person is re-experiencing trauma in what could be described as a state of partial arousal. The episodes could be conceptualized as simultaneous re-experiencing and reworking of trauma. Freud referred to this particular process as "abreaction". The episodes tend to be paroxysmal in nature, i.e. they have an abrupt and unexpected onset. In addition to being intrusive, the episodes are also recurrent. They are recurrent, because it is difficult to achieve full resolution of the traumatic memory and traumatic affects on a single occasion.

Integration and resolution of traumatic events are, in the majority of cases, a process rather than a single event. The nature of the experience may be so threatening that it is impossible to absorb and integrate on a single occasion. Instead, the processing of trauma is distributed over a period of time and takes place through multiple abreactive episodes. In each one of these episodes, the traumatic experience is remobilized, i.e. it is brought into awareness in a piecemeal fashion.

The processing or integration of traumatic experience resembles, to some extent, the management of liquids which are stored in a tank under pressure. Substances stored in such a way require special handling. A little bit is let out at a time through a mechanism, usually a valve, which permits control over what could otherwise result in flooding.

Dynamic functions of pseudoseizures

Drawing from a variety of observations concerning the nature of the post-traumatic response, especially some recurrent challenges which traumatized individuals tend to be confronted with, we might summarize the functions of pseudoseizures as follows:

A large proportion of pseudoseizures represent a response to a traumatic experience.

They do not arise at random and they play a role in the process of coping with that experience. Their primary functions are:

- Pseudoseizures represent a defense against re-experiencing trauma in an overwhelming way. They are a defense against collapse of personality and affective flooding.
- Pseudoseizure episodes can also represent partial re-experiencing and partial reworking of trauma where traumatic experience is of such a nature that it cannot be dealt with on a single occasion. Thus, pseudoseizures are both a symptom of trauma, and an attempt at solution. They can be viewed as a mechanism which combines simultaneous remobilization and working through of trauma.
- Pseudoseizures can serve as a powerful defense against anger which is evoked in response to trauma, or specifically anger against the aggressor. In that context, the person would rather suffer than lose control of anger and hurt someone else.
- Pseudoseizures can also represent a defense against narcissistic injuries.

The four functions are complimentary. In a given patient, at a given time, one function may be of particular significance, and may play a dominant role. However, a capacity to serve multiple psychodynamic goals is probably one of the reasons why pseudoseizures are frequent in post-traumatic settings and also why they tend to be persistent.

Special topics in treatment of traumatic conditions

Topics reviewed in this section deal with issues which may arise in the course of treatment of traumatized individuals, including pseudoseizure patients. These issues have to do with processing of difficult affects and memories. The therapeutic challenge inherent in this task can be made easier if the clinician appreciates the psychodynamic significance of those processes.

Contents of another time

Traumatized individuals frequently experience persistent intrusive recollections of people or events related to the trauma. The complexity and intensity of the remembered material vary considerably.

The remembered material is not simply a memory. It is certainly not a memory in the sense that remembering where one put one's keys is a memory. Rather, this material typically includes complex traumatic affect—frequently a mixture of dysphoria, agitation, and anger.

The most acute and intense form of traumatic remembering is a flashback which is considered a hallmark of the post-traumatic stress disorder (PTSD). Flashbacks, however, do not occur in all post-traumatic reactions and they may be absent in chronic cases. The person could, nevertheless, be troubled by a persistent intrusion of the past traumatic experience and its associated affects. This essentially amounts to reliving the past, on a more or less regular basis, while trying to live in the present as well.

Traumatic intrusions of this kind were described by Freud (1917, in "Mourning and Melancholia") as occurring in complicated mourning, and were, in fact, considered as a characteristic trajectory of reactions to traumatic loss.

Many post-traumatic reactions contain a component of complicated mourning, and they follow the path of complicated mourning which is characterized by this intrusive emergence of the past into the baseline of present experience.

In a sense, the patient feels emotionally compelled to live his daily life on two timelines or two schedules. Part of the time, he lives as if the past were happening now. He or she is not merely dwelling on the past. Dwelling on the past implies chiefly thinking about it a good deal.

Being trapped emotionally in two timelines is a psychologically much more difficult process as it contains the intense affective pull in which the affects of the past not only intrude themselves into the present affective baseline but begin to pervade it.

This psychological situation is characterized by an intense competition between two psychological processes. One orients the person towards the present and things that matter in the present. The other process drives the person into remobilizing past experience and its affects, over and over, until they are integrated. This process of living on two timelines is very painful and psychologically costly. It represents more than just a present into which a few bad memories are scattered. It really amounts to substantial energies of the personality being shunted away from their proper focus of dealing with the present.

As unpleasant as it may seem, and as futile as it may seem, this process is not really self-defeating although it may appear so to the outsiders.

Re-mobilization of past experience is not a voluntary, conscious action or a decision on the part of the person to "live in the past". There is an automatic, or even compulsive quality about this process. It is a form of compulsory emotional remembering which the person does not really choose to engage in. It represents an attempt to gradually desensitize the person of the intense traumatic charge which their memories carry.

Trauma victims, especially veterans with PTSD, in whom this process of ongoing entanglement with their traumatic past is very evident, are often a focus of criticism by others who see them as engaging in something unproductive, or, worse yet, self-indulgent. This criticism is often accompanied by the belief that the traumatized individual is choosing to live in the past, and that they have a full, indeed, perfect control over their affective state which they could get out of easily, if only they put their mind to it.

While it is true that some traumatized individuals respond in unproductive and self-indulgent ways, the primary reason for compulsive emotional remembering of the past is not self-indulgence. It is also not unproductive, or rather, it is not only unproductive. It is true that it is unproductive with respect to someone's current goals or keeping one's current life going. This goal however, is not the only psychological task the traumatized individual is facing. He or she is compelled to address the disrupted psychological balance which trauma inevitably causes. This disruption requires that the traumatic experience be processed until it has been—somehow—integrated.

The individual is thus under psychological pressure to own all and not just some of the experience which he or she has encountered. Thus, one is not so much dwelling on the past as trying to keep faith with the past, in order to maintain a sense of closure and wholeness.

The drive to maintain closure and wholeness is no less important than the pleasure/pain principle, and, in traumatic states, this drive is directly at odds with the pleasure/pain principle. As the pleasure/pain principle and the drive toward wholeness are two major axes along which personality functioning is organized, their conflict is psychologically costly. This particular conflict accounts for a good deal of complexity of post-traumatic adaptation. Post-traumatic adaptation often makes no sense if we attempt to account for it solely in terms of pleasure/pain principle.

Traumatized individuals who are entangled with their disturbing memories live their lives as though their day were divisible—part of it is for the past and part of it is for the present. This is not because they lack a conscious appreciation of the fact that it would be far better for them if they could invest all their energies into their present goals. To tell them that they are dwelling in the past is not telling them anything they don't already know. They know it all too well.

Their situation could be compared to the situation of a builder who in the process of building a house discovers that the foundation of the house has cracked. He is obliged to repair the rift in the foundation before he ventures on to complete the top stories of the house.

Reworking the past by re-mobilizing it, albeit in traumatic ways, is thus not a self-defeating process, but something one is obliged to deal with before moving on. This does not mean that traumatized individuals caught in the midst of this process are not experiencing significant pain or disruption, even immobilization. Depending on the severity of symptoms accompanying intrusive remembering of the past, therapeutic modalities other than outpatient therapy may be required (medication, even hospitalization).

This disruption cannot be completely avoided. Nevertheless, understanding that this process, which has a very eruptive, spasmodic and capricious quality, is, in fact, not a way of failing, but a way of reworking and mastering the trauma, is helpful for both the therapist and the patient.

How to handle the compulsive need to ventilate

A certain proportion of acutely traumatized individuals, or therapy patients who are in the process of acute reactivation of the trauma feel a compulsive need to ventilate. This process can take on an almost autonomous quality. The patient continues to be anxious while ventilating, thus giving the appearance that no relief is actually in sight, and that the therapeutic process is becoming stalled. On the other hand, the patient resists efforts to be diverted and, in response to them, becomes even more anxious or insistent.

The driven quality of this process, combined with the fact that it is repeated over and over, with no net gain, can be baffling to the therapist or some other individual who is trying to help. Eventually, the therapist will need to make a decision as to how and when to take charge of this process and redirect the patient. This is a technical issue which various therapists handle in different ways, depending on how they understand the patient's situation, their individual therapeutic style, etc. We cannot speak of one and only one accurate method of achieving this challenging yet necessary transition in therapy, but, rather, of *different* accurate methods.

At some point in this process, the therapist may begin to experience the traumatic material and the patient's urgency and intensity as disturbing. This response on the part of the therapist/or other clinician is by no means blameworthy. Such a response is natural and understandable, and is a legitimate problem of therapists who deal with traumatized populations. How to remain helpful and useful to the patient in spite of these feelings is an important goal of training, in fact, it is one of the most significant professional achievements. Being disturbed by the patient's affective urgency can occur in spite of excellent professional skill and experience, however. It is important that the therapist conceptualize this situation as any other therapeutic challenge, and not as a sign of inadequacy, either on his part or the patient's.

Situations of this kind can trigger in the therapist a fear that he or she will not be able to contain the patient's agitation at all, and that this particular failure, in turn, will inevitably lead to the breakdown of the whole therapeutic enterprise. This fear is frequently accompanied by a sense of shame, and anticipation that this particular patient will expose the therapist as a failure.

When faced with such affects in himself the therapist should initiate attempts at self-soothing, just as he (or she) would attempt to reassure another person.

The following point of view might be considered:

While I am experiencing this patient as a threat, he or she is not, or, not necessarily, acting this way IN ORDER to be a threat to me. The situation we are facing now is not a test of the patient's worth or mine. Although I feel very anxious, it is not my fault, nor is it the patient's fault. And although I don't really understand this, nor can I help the patient's feelings go away right now, I may, eventually, and that is good enough.

After achieving some measure of composure, the therapist may proceed to reassure the patient:

I can see how difficult it must be to have to face something which makes you feel like you cannot get a hold of it no matter how hard you try.

OR

I appreciate how hard it must be to feel that you may not be able to get rid of this feeling, no matter how hard you work.

OR

I realize that you are very afraid of (or concerned with) what might happen if you are not able to solve this whole situation right now.

OR

I realize that you are very afraid that you may not be able to manage if you are not able to make yourself feel better right away (what will happen to you if you cannot make yourself better right now).

Although we may not be able to make it all completely better for you right now, in time, we may. Right now, you are only responsible for the next step which is your next appointment.

You have already done a responsible thing by coming here.— Between now and your next appointment you needn't do anything special, just perhaps begin to pace yourself because I will need your help again when we next meet.

Select contributions from object-relations theory

Psychological security and early experience

A great deal of clinical evidence supports the view that psychological security of an individual throughout life is intimately tied to the nature of his or her early experience of nurturance. While the role of the mother (or primary caretaker) is widely understood to be of greatest significance, it is not always easy to specify how nurturance translates into emotional security. Nurturance is often assumed to be a simple and self-evident process and its role in the development of emotional security equally self-evident.

Clinical investigators and theorists who deal with the nature of attachment, however, have shown that, far from being a single entity, attachment is a process, a very elaborate process in the course of which different aspects of emotional maturation are mastered at different stages. And conversely, failure to master certain emotional skills at the appropriate stage is associated with vulnerability to developing certain psychological difficulties and symptoms. Thus, emotional development is a process in which, at critical junctures, one either progresses towards a desirable goal, or one regresses to an earlier (which often means no longer appropriate) form of emotional interaction and expression. In that sense, the developing child does not really have the option of standing still, i.e. of not dealing with the age-appropriate emotional challenges, any more than a person who is in the ocean has the option not to swim. Maturation of emotional ties thus has an inherent potential to be disruptive, with resolution occurring often through the medium of conflict, rather than by a smooth transition from stage to stage.

The nature of the maternal role, as it pertains to the subsequent development of emotional stability and security, can perhaps be best understood by focusing on her actual functions. During the better part of the first year her role is quite comprehensive. She has the responsibility not only for the infant's physical needs and comfort, but also to ensure that his daily environment is so well controlled that the sources of stimulation which impinge on the infant are not excessive, but are optimal. In a sense, she modulates and conditions the child's environment. This particular aspect of the mother's role as a psychological shield was emphasized by several attachment theorists.

W. R. Bion

Bion (1977) made significant contributions to our understanding of the very early, preverbal phases of personality development. He emphasized the importance of the mother as a psychic container for the infant's physical tensions and intense or disorganized affect. He felt that the infant, due to his immaturity, was particularly liable to experiencing frequent discomfort arising from bodily needs or external environment and that discomfort (from a variety of sources) could promptly translate into intense emotional reactions and overwhelming fears. Thus, from the point of view of the child's experience, there is but a minimal distance between hunger or being wet to the psychological experience of impending catastrophe.

Because of this extreme way of processing the internal and external stimulation (which from the child's point of view could not be readily differentiated), there is a clear need for the maternal role of stimulus filtering. She serves as the child's stimulus barrier. Not only does she have the role of a sensory barrier, but she, in her function as a container, has a specific role of "detoxifying" his physical tension states and overwhelming or disorganized affect (Bion, 1977).

Detoxificaton is achieved because the mother responds to the infant's disorganized state in a particular way, namely by empathy, attunement, and of particular significance, by being willing to receive his painful states (to be a container) without being emotionally threatened by them. Bion postulated this process whereby the mother essentially serves as a depository of the child's bad internal experience and in doing so changes the nature of those experiences, as being critical to developing a sense of emotional safety. The child projects onto her his bad experience, which is then "modified by the container so that the infant may take it back into its own personality in a tolerable form" (Bion, 1977, p. 27).

D. W. Winnicott

The role of the mother as someone who protects the infant from environmental overstimulation was also emphasized by Winnicott who referred to it as the "holding function". He defined this aspects of nurturance in the following manner: "The holding environment therefore has as its main function the reduction to a minimum of impingements to which the infant must react with resultant annihilation of personal being" (Winnicott, 1965, p. 47). He further states that, "anxiety in these early stages of parent-infant relationship relates to the threat of annihilation" (p. 47). This observation of Winnicott's in which he links the excessive stimulation by the environment to annihilation anxiety in an immature system is one of his important contributions as the connection is by no means obvious. Thus, the mother is conceptualized as playing a very active role in holding all adverse or excessive or irrelevant parts of the environment at bay.

Margaret Mahler

On the basis of extensive observations of mother/infant and mother/child interactions in the course of the first four years of life, Margaret Mahler evolved an elaborate theory of attachment as it progresses through a number of distinct phases. Each of these stages requires that the child face a different task of emotional development. According to Mahler, emotional development progresses from a stage in which the child is psychologically inseparable from the mother (symbiotic phase) through various intermediate stages in which he gradually gains greater emotional autonomy, towards the stage at which he can achieve a balance between neediness and independence.

Emotional independence is a concept which is much more difficult to define than physical independence. It is not a single entity, but rather a composite of different emotional assets or abilities. Also, it is not directly observable; rather, its presence can be inferred from a variety of diverse indicators.

Emotional independence is a significant aspect of emotional maturity. Its chief component is the ability to regulate one's mood and self esteem, without having to evoke support from another person. While support from another person is a natural aspect of social life on which people rely routinely, compulsive neediness and reliance on others to regulate one's psychological well-being is a form of excessive psychological dependence.

The opposite of dependence is a state of having individuated. Margaret Mahler thus conceptualized the process of attainment of emotional maturity as one of achieving an optimal level of individuation (Mahler, 1968).

Mahler conceptualized the processes of individuation as a crucial component of the "psychological birth" of the individual. Individuation essentially, refers to the very gradual growth of a person's ability to regulate himself psychologically without having to manipulate or coerce other people or merge with them psychologically. This process is intimately connected with mood and aspects of close relationships which relate specifically to the satisfaction of emotional needs.

The initial stage of the process of psychological birth is referred to by Mahler as "normal autism" (Mahler, 1968). It includes the first month of life. During this period there is virtually no recognition, on the infant's part, of the mother as a separate being. He is not able to differentiate satisfaction of needs which occurs as a result of his mother's efforts from his own measures at reducing tension. In this highly undifferentiated state, he is only aware of the quality of experience as such—either good or bad, pleasurable or painful-regardless of how this state was achieved. Psychologically speaking, the infant functions, as if he were in his own "autistic orbit" and "need satisfaction belongs to his own omnipotent autistic orbit"(p. 8).

During the second month the child's psychological experience changes with a beginning awareness of the mother as "a need-satisfying object" (p. 8). Mahler refers to this new phase as "normal symbiosis".

During the symbiotic phase "the infant behaves and functions as though he and his mother were an omnipotent system – a dual unity within one common boundary" (p. 8).

This rudimentary form of psychological relatedness has several important characteristics. Because of the child's immaturity, the mother provides a homeostatic function—she regulates his experience and emotional processing for him. She volunteers her own psychological resources to manage his world. Through her ongoing, very focused ministrations, she ensures tension reduction, and also provides a buffering function from all environmental stimuli that are irrelevant. Mahler shares with Winnicott and Bion the recognition of the importance of the maternal psychological buffering as an instrument of emotional growth.

Symbiotic attachment thus provides a "safe anchorage" for the child (Mahler, 1968, p. 17). It has also been described as a "smoothly balanced" relationship in which "the infant fundamentally has the security that his needs will be met without having to recognize his dependency upon an external object for survival" (Giovacchini, 1976, p. 420, cited by Sperling in Fine, 1989, p. 359). This is a particularly powerful aspect of symbiotic attachment—it presumes an intuitive and implicit understanding of one's needs on the part of the mother. The feeling accompanying this state in which all needs are met automatically and as matter of course is one of omnipotence (the corollary to the infant's sense of omnipotence is his perception that the mother is likewise omnipotent).

Following the period of symbiotic attachment, the infant begins the process of "breaking away, in a bodily sense, from his hitherto completely passive lap-babyhood" by his tentative efforts to explore his surroundings (Mahler, 1972). Mahler called this initial stage of emotional differentiation—"hatching". This transitional state gives way to the phase called "practicing" which is characterized by the maturation of motor function which permits the child much greater confidence in exploring his environment. The freedom to explore is often accompanied by a sense of exuberance, a feeling that "the world is his oyster". Mahler noted that children in this subphase show considerable tolerance for frustration, a certain "imperviousness". The sense of exuberance serves as an affective shield against frustration .The mother's role at this stage is to accept and foster his growing attempts at separation—a role which is considerably different from her earlier role of providing massive psychological buttressing.

The period of practicing is superseded by the rapprochement phase (spanning the period from 15 to 22 months). This phase is psychologically much more complex, because the child begins to sense that his needs will no longer be fulfilled implicitly and automatically, that the mother is a person with her own needs, and that her needs and his no longer coincide. This is not a conscious insight, but a stressful feeling which begins to invade his daily experience and which is gradually crystallized from a number of interactions in which his expectations for mother's availability were not met.

The notion that our needs will not be met by others implicitly seems self-evident—almost axiomatic—a social given that every reasonable human being is expected to live by. Mahler's observations of children's development, however, indicate that the acceptance of emotional separateness of others is anything but a simple matter. This acceptance is not easily come by. Quite the contrary, it is a major achievement and a major milestone in the personality/emotional development. It is a difficult psychological achievement which has to be negotiated through the rapprochement conflict.

From the point of view of the rapprochement child, the growing awareness that one no longer lives protected within a magical union is a painful psychological transition. However, this form of emotional separation is crucial to achieve before the child can individuate. Still, the awareness of the mother (and later, other significant people)—as separate psychological beings- is infinitely more difficult to tolerate than the awareness of her as a separate physical entity. The latter is a cognitive achievement which is accomplished without any emotional cost to the child. By contrast, psychological separateness of others, particularly significant others, is initiated through a rude awakening.

Separateness really means that one no longer has a safe anchorage in another person and that, furthermore, this loss occurred capriciously, for no good reason and through no fault of our own. Thus, the process of individuation at the rapprochement stage is initiated through traumatic awareness that, emotionally, one cannot assume certain things which were implicitly there only recently and which we therefore came to regard as our right, i.e. others do not belong to us emotionally as a matter of course.

Mahler writes (1972, p. 494):

> It has already begun to dawn on the junior toddler that the world is not his oyster; that he must cope with it more or less on his own, very often as a relatively helpless, small and separate individual, unable to command relief and assistance merely by feeling the need for them or giving voice to that need.

The awareness of separateness of others really amounts to a realization that their sustaining presence can no longer be taken for granted. It is not a neutral event. This awareness is accompanied by considerable separation anxiety which the child tries to contain by urgent efforts to reconnect with the mother—a behavior which Mahler called "shadowing".

During the rapprochement phase a child is torn between two opposing emotional pulls. On the one hand, there is the regressive pull towards reestablishing a safe emotional anchorage with the mother on the symbiotic basis (which is, however, no longer developmentally appropriate). This is a form of emotional merging. As natural as that yearning for a merger is, it does not really provide a solution for a child in his second or third year, because it does not meet his other developmental needs for a vigorous mastery of his world which can only occur by embracing his surroundings.

The child at this stage is thus forced to find a compromise between divergent emotional needs and ways of relating. One of them is a longing for an all-nurturing presence. The other is an equally strong pressure to gain self-efficacy and self-definition through many exchanges with the environment in which one's abilities are tested (the rapprochement crisis).

The challenge of the rapprochement phase—which is also the major challenge of individuation—is having to deal not so much with the physical absence of the mother, as with the sudden and unanticipated loss of her as a sustaining presence.

The optimal response on the mother's part during this stage is to be "quietly available" (Mahler, 1972, p. 495). This means that she will permit the child a good measure of independence, so that he does not feel constrained in undertaking new tasks in discovering his surroundings. On the other hand, she is emotionally available when he seeks to reconnect with her, and allows him to choose the terms on which he wants to reconnect.

This is, in many ways, an ideal way of relating which, however, requires a great deal of sensitivity on the mother's part. To be "quietly available" means that she is neither intrusive nor withholding with respect to the child. However, in order to achieve this balance between distance and availability she is required to maintain a state of ongoing concern and attunement which really amounts to emotional vigilance without action. The quiet availability is thus emotionally very demanding and anything but a passive process. To remain connected without infringing on another person requires a good deal of emotional security, maturity and sensitivity (an optimal maternal, as well as therapeutic stance).

The optimal approach on the mother's part thus includes a combination of two distinct emotional responses: (1) her enthusiastic support for the child's undertakings, i.e. for projects he undertakes on his own initiative and (2) being reliably emotionally available when he seeks her out.

A combination of these two emotional attitudes or reactions has an inherently therapeutic value, and not just for children. However, for children at this crucial stage, this particular way of being nurturing helps to develop a range of feelings which go beyond the brittle extremes of union, on the one hand, and catastrophic loss on the other. The child gradually acquires an intermediate range of affect and relatedness.

Once acquired, this intermediate range serves as a substantive protection against panic and emptiness (i.e. it constitutes an internal structure). It helps consolidate a belief in a benign world—a sense that one will not be catastrophically abandoned if one ventures into the world which beckons to him. This is major achievement of emotional adaptation.

If the child who is attempting to individuate is not supported in his efforts and the mother withdraws her emotional support whenever he seeks out autonomy, an intense crisis can be precipitated, because the child will sense that he must give up his sense of identity and efficacy if he means to keep his mother's sustaining love. That conflict will activate intense efforts to bring the mother back. From the child's point of view, he needs to get her back at any cost. So much effort will be spent in accomplishing this task, that the child's energy might be diverted from those developmental tasks in other domains of his life, which are equally important for his or her sense of well-being.

A question arises as to why the realization that the mother is a separate being—that she no longer responds to everything the child feels, as he feels it, and is no longer an all-sustaining presence—would be so traumatic.

From the adult's point of view, the idea that the fulfillment of needs is something which is negotiated (even if not formally) with another person is not striking. From the point of view of a two- or three-year-old child, however, the sudden or even gradual withdrawal of emotional supplies can be nothing short of catastrophic—he has no basis for knowing that it is not permanent. He does not have cognitive or emotional resources to experience it as a reversible emotional setback. Rather, he experiences it as an emotional wall between himself and the mother which has appeared for no reason. At this stage of affective development, he does not have the capacity to grasp provisional realities (temporary setback, temporary loss), only extremes. The withdrawal of the mother as an all-sustaining presence appears to him *entirely arbitrary as well as permanent*.

The rapprochement child cannot really be certain that maternal unavailability in one situation does not, like a domino, imply she will never again be available, or that her failure to meet a small need does not imply that she will abandon him in an emergency. The only way he can resolve this painful doubt is experientially, which means that he (or she) has to be able to tolerate anxiety which accompanies risk-taking. He needs to be independent for a while, and then return to the fold to find that the mother—as a nurturing presence, not just as a physical being—is still there. This process needs to be repeated over and over until the child learns, to his satisfaction, that the mother's absence is not permanent, and that he can therefore tolerate it.

From being repeatedly separated and reunited, he also begins to learn to negotiate emotional distance and closeness in a relationship. This eventually contributes to the development of a sense of assurance that one can be emotionally safe even without symbiotic attachment.

If, on the other hand, he does not acquire this rudimentary emotional security (i.e. if the rapprochement crisis has an unfavorable outcome), the child's internalized experience of mothering or nurturance will be highly polarized, i.e. reduced to extremes. When he merges with her psychologically he will feel good about her and about himself. On the other hand, when he ventures on his own and his primary concern is to engage the world and not to respond to her, or relate to her, he will feel that he is bad and that she is bad (as a result of the internalized maternal disapproval.) In a sense, he will feel bad not just whenever he takes initiative, but worse yet, because he took the initiative. This means that he will feel guilty about his own sense of agency.

A sense of agency is a psychological experience of being able to initiate things that keep one engaged with the world, and able to keep pace with the world through one's own efforts. The sense of agency is naturally accompanied by confidence and pleasure. The opposite of the sense of agency is a state in which one is stalled in one's own fear, and rather than initiating action, is stung into action by the world's many provoking causes. This state is frequently accompanied by feelings of guilt and inadequacy.

In reviewing Mahler's contributions to our understanding of the dynamics of attachment, it should be borne in mind that she is not dealing with concrete entities or even single ideas. She is studying what we might loosely call emotional skills although that term too is not really adequate. A skill usually implies something which is largely (although not inevitably) in the domain of conscious thought and is taught in a much more straightforward and direct way, with clear feedback for success and failure. None of this is really true of complex emotional growth. Early attachment is not a single process, but rather, a field of experience and action. A good deal of what happens in that field cannot be easily articulated, especially not in verbal terms. Mahler's designations of symbiosis, practicing, hatching etc, are not so much clinical terms as they are her attempts to capture the emotional truth of the major developmental phases, as she came to understand them through intensive observation and through dynamic intuitive links.

She conceptualized attachment as a dynamic process in which something develops only through an ongoing interaction between two individuals, in this instance, mother and child. Thus, she deals with emotional growth as it occurs through an ongoing exchange of emotional experience. It would not be surprising to discover that such a form of learning would be very laborious. The ongoing interaction is eventually internalized, leading to a development of more or less stable inner structures—psychic structures which reflect the affective quality of interaction between mother and child—that which has been absorbed and assimilated.

Like all internalized material, a psychic structure is not a replica or a conscious memory of an event or a person. Rather, it represents a distillate of many repeated interactions, in particular, their emotional tone. The emotional tone is remembered *the way taste or sound is remembered.* These internalized summaries of our early attachment history and our early sense of self have been called internal objects and the theory which deals with them *object-relations theory*. The "object" in this context refers to an internalized representation of an important relationship.

As we noted earlier, the internal representation is not a concept or a memory, rather it is a piece of our emotional history which serves as a guide to future emotional relationships. Its essential characteristic is that it evokes feelings. If the feelings it evokes are good (a good internal object or introject), then we meet new relationships with confidence and pleasurable anticipation. If the feelings are painful (a hostile internal object or introject) then we meet new attachments with anxiety, ambivalence and insecurity.

Internal objects are thus emotional signposts which help us navigate the emotional and social world. They form a matrix of our emotional/interpersonal experience—defined by pleasure or pain—as it relates to our ties with others. They contain instrumentalities of nurturance: on what terms and with what emotional consequences or cost we can expect to have our needs fulfilled by others.

Object-relations theory and borderline syndromes

The object-relations approach is not a single theoretical system. It contains a number of distinct theories which elucidate different aspects of personality and affective development. It offers accounts of normal development; however, its particular emphasis is on pathological developments. Contributions of various object-relations theorists are especially important in dealing with the complexities of borderline syndromes as they offer a conceptual framework for approaching this disorder.

The term "borderline syndromes" encompasses diverse clinical presentations. Some of them conform to the diagnosis of the "borderline personality disorder" as defined by the fourth edition of the Diagnostic and Statistical Manual of Mental Disorders (DSM-IV, American Psychiatric Association, 1994, pp. 650–54). Various partial presentations, however, are also frequently encountered. Thus, the term "borderline syndromes" may include, but is not limited to the borderline personality disorder.

I am concerned here with the borderline syndromes, because it is my contention that trauma, especially chronic trauma, might generate clinical presentations which strongly resemble borderline syndromes. Indeed, I maintain that an important subset of post-traumatic syndromes closely resembles borderline syndromes.

I further maintain that one might conceptualize borderline syndromes as a form of *regression* in the overall personality functioning which occurs as a result of trauma. This means that a person who has experienced trauma, which is sufficiently intense or sufficiently chronic, may regress to a borderline level of functioning without being a borderline personality disorder.

A certain proportion of pseudoseizure patients have a clinical presentation which resembles borderline syndromes, especially traumatically induced borderline syndromes. For this reason, it is important to become familiar with key psychodynamic concepts which elucidate characteristic features of affect, relatedness and attachment found in this challenging disorder.

Borderline syndromes are complex, both from the standpoint of their clinical presentations, as well as theoretically. A great variety of symptoms often occur in borderline cases, typically including some mixture of depressive symptomatology and anxiety. Of particular concern are intense and unstable interpersonal relationships, as well as problems with impulse control (the latter, while quite intense, need not occur in every case).

The clinical presentation is challenging for several reasons. The first has to do with the variability and intensity of the symptoms. The second reason has to do with symptoms not fitting traditional neurotic or psychotic patterns.

Object-relations theorists have argued that these patients are not merely exhibiting a variety of symptoms, but are organized on a level that differs qualitatively from both neurotic and psychotic presentations. In other words, they are structurally different.

A full account of the psychodynamics of the borderline syndromes is beyond the scope of this work and will not be attempted in this context. However, we shall draw selectively from the wealth of observations and focus specifically on those concepts which are most relevant and most helpful in understanding characteristic relational pathology and regressed affective states, as these issues are most troublesome to patients and therapists alike.

As will be recalled from our earlier discussion, object-relations theorists conceptualize affective and personality development in terms of structural units which are referred to as object-relations units. These units are templates which contain significant emotional information about relationships with people who are responsible for nurturing the child and are critically important in his early development. An object-relations unit is not a single memory or feeling or experience – it is composed of accumulated memories and feelings and experiences. It is a composite within which is organized a rudimentary sense of self, a rudimentary sense of what others are, and a feeling tone—either pleasure or displeasure—which typically accompanied being with another-person (Kernberg, 1976).

Otto Kernberg

Kernberg is one of the theoretical and treatment pioneers whose work has helped to define the object-relations approach to borderline syndromes. Out of his comprehensive treatment of this subject we shall present key features of early object-relations development.

Kernberg conceptualized the maturation of affect and maturation of the sense of self as proceeding along two pathways: toward greater differentiation and toward greater integration (or stabilization).

The rudimentary units develop as a consolidation of affective experience, either positive or negative. As a result of gratifying, pleasurable interactions with the mother, an object-relations unit develops which is permeated with positive affect. This early unit contains rudimentary images of self, as well as rudimentary images of others. Initially, the sense of self is indistinguishable from the sense of others, but gradually, a sense of self becomes more defined (Kernberg, 1976, p. 61).

As a counterpart to the object-relations unit which is dominated by pleasurable affect, there develops, as a consequence of consolidation of negative and painful interactions (when needs are not met)—the "bad" primary intrapsychic structure (p. 61). Within this structure as well, the boundary between the experience of self and the sense of others is initially obscure, but becomes increasingly distinct later (p. 61). Being able to achieve this differentiation is one of the critical tasks of early development (failure to achieve it leads to psychotic vulnerability, p. 60).

In discussing object-relations units, it should be noted that they are not ideas—although they give rise to the ideas and are elaborated through ideas. They are primarily consolidated affective memories of being with others—either feeling good and safe or feeling threatened and abandoned.

The rudimentary structures discussed above are known as "partial self-object units", because they precede the development of a fully integrated sense of self and others. In order for this to occur, the next important developmental stage has to be completed. This stage entails *integration* of partial self-object relations units (p. 64). As noted earlier, these partial units are primarily affective constellations—either positively toned or negatively toned. At the beginning of this new stage, the sense of self is still split between the "good me" and the "bad me". Likewise, the sense of others is experienced through extremes which are either exclusively positive ("good object") or exclusively negative ("bad object"). In order to develop a stable personality organization, it is critical to be able to integrate these primitive affective extremes into a coherent sense of self, as well as a coherent sense of others.

The above account of the formation of personality structure is complex and has several important implications. To begin with, it implies that the personality and the awareness of self emerge from affect and that the earliest foundation of the sense of self is really affect. Thus, affect is the earliest experience and the earliest orientation to the world.

Initially, this affect consists of crude extremes—safety as opposed to threat—feeling good or feeling bad. The sense of feeling good/bad precedes the awareness of the world and the awareness of oneself. This implies that, in these very early stages, the sense of self and the sense of the world barely exist independently. Rather, they are enmeshed or imbedded in this matrix of feeling. Consequently, they are quite fragile, and scarcely have any independent existence, and can change rapidly as the affect changes. Thus, how we see ourselves and how we perceive others to whom we are meant to relate is powerfully influenced by the affective surround, by the climate of affect. Clearly, this early world is not determined by ideas, but by the primitive sense of safety and threat within which our sense of self is tentatively established.

Thus, the sense of self (and the other) is initially critically dependent on affect. We might say that the sense of self is ushered in by affect, especially affects of union and well-being.

Object-relations theorists are especially interested in this critical dependence and its implications for later personality development. Specifically, they have noted that, in borderline syndromes, the patients readily regress to the stage where the sense of self and the sense of others is driven by or entrained by developmentally earlier affective states and modes of relatedness which implies (among other things) that the patients can only experience themselves and others in terms of affective extremes.

Masterson and Rinsley

Masterson and Rinsley have made further contributions to our understanding of the dynamics of borderline syndromes by elaborating the complexities of the rapprochement struggle in borderline patients (recall earlier discussion of rapprochement phase in Mahler). They noted the role of the borderline mother as one of the important factors contributing to the pathological outcome of the rapprochement crisis. In addition, they have elaborated the nature of internal experience which characterizes borderline patients.

According to Masterson (Masterson, in Grotstein, 1987, p. 208):

> The borderline mother, unable to separate fully from her own mother, clings to her child and fosters the symbiotic relationship to maintain her own intrapsychic equilibrium. She is unable to deal with the child's emerging separation-individuation as it interrupts her clinging and exposes her to separation anxiety.

Because of the anxiety evoked in her by the child's effort to strike out on his own, she does not support sufficiently his increasing curiosity and assertiveness which normally characterize the rapprochement phase. "She is available if the child clings and behaves regressively, but withdraws from his efforts to separate and individuate". (Masterson, in Grotstein, 1987, p. 208).

As a consequence of this particular response to the child's need to become more independent, the child finds himself in a peculiar bind—he can only be loved and responded to when he clings or fuses emotionally, i.e. as long as he does nothing to remind his mother that he is a separate person. This, in turn, deprives him of a great deal of normal and expected experimentation and exploration of the environment. Since the child cannot stop his efforts to be more independent, he will encounter rejection. Their relationship assumes a "push-pull quality" (Rinsley, in Hartcollis, 1977, p. 56).

The notion that the child can be loved only when he clings or fuses emotionally implies that the child will be vulnerable to regression when he encounters rejection. Vulnerability to regression, in turn, is one of the difficulties which are especially characteristic of the interpersonal predicament of borderline individuals.

The highly conflicted way in which the nurturance and support are given to the child is very disruptive. What the child internalizes, as a result of the particular terms on which nurturance is provided, is likewise disrupted and conflicted. Instead of internalizing a consistently positive emotional tone related to a close relationship, he or she will internalize one which is highly polarized and therefore unstable.

Masterson and Rinsley (Rinsley, in Hartcollis, 1977, p. 58) have conceptualized the internalized experience of mother-child interactions as consisting of two parts. The first is called the *rewarding* (*libidinal*) *part unit*. This unit represents a remnant or distillate of gratifying and sustaining interactions which occurred when the mother was emotionally available. However, that availability was dependent on the child behaving in a regressive and clinging way. The internalized emotional experience which comprises the rewarding unit contains several components. The first is the internalized image of the mother associated with approval, support and nurturance. This image of the mother is emotionally linked with the image of oneself as being good, albeit a passive child. The affective tone of the rewarding unit is highly positive.

The second part of the internalized unit has entirely opposite qualities, in fact, it is drastically different. It is referred to as the *withdrawing* (*rejecting, aggressive*) *part unit*. The mother is internalized as "attacking, critical, hostile, angry, withdrawing or withholding supplies and approval in the face of assertiveness or other efforts toward separation-individuation" (Rinsley in Hartcollis, 1977, p. 58). The image of the self, which corresponds to this experience of the mother, is being bad, helpless, evil or empty. The affective tone associated with this unit is a combination of chronic anger and abandonment depression.

The model evolved by Masterson and Rinsley underscores the complexity and the compelling nature of the self-experience and experience of others which occurs during this particular developmental crisis in children who later become borderline adults.

The internalized experience which exists in terms of the withdrawing or rewarding object-relations units has several characteristics .It is a tense and unstable system. The affective constellations involved are very powerful and they allow very little emotional flexibility. In many ways, they remind one of the world of a medieval legend—the good are very good and the bad are very bad.

It should be added, in this context, that the borderline individual (when under the impact of the withdrawing/rejecting constellation) does not believe that others are truly persecuting him. His experience is not based on delusional beliefs – he is not truly paranoid. His sense of threat does not stem from a thought disorder, but from a feeling state which, while it lasts, is very compelling and seems totally natural to him. He acts and feels *as if* he were threatened.

The withdrawing/rewarding constellations are both overly intense and too simple to provide reliable orientation in interpersonal relationships. They are not a reasoned response to a clearly understood situation, or to another person as they really are. Rather, they could be compared to fixed action patterns. This is a term which ethologists, i.e. scientists who deal with animal behavior, use to describe units of action which, once set in motion, are typically carried out to completion, and are not responsive to ongoing circumstances nor can they be readily inhibited. The units are highly instinctual and stereotypic. The animal behavior is, to some extent, composed of these units. They are important and adaptive when simple actions are called for, as it would be far too dangerous to be obliged to invent a new method of dealing with a particular danger every time one encountered it.

In attempting to describe the nature of behavior which is characteristic of a fixed action pattern, the author is reminded of an event which actually took place in her house. A young sparrow flew into a room adjoining the garden by mistake. It was still very young and just learning to fly. The sparrow became promptly alarmed and made vigorous attempts to get out. However, it could only fly in a straight line, back and forth, in the same vertical plane. This line closely paralleled one of the glass walls. Knowing that the bird would be very frightened of any attempt to catch it, I took advantage of a bouquet of gladioli which was on the table and offered one of them to the sparrow. The gladiolus, measuring about two and a half feet, seemed an ideal bridge. To my surprise, the sparrow just kept flying – in the same plane – past the gladiolus. It was unable to make use of the gladiolus, because the flower was slightly off to the side of the plane in which it was flying. It was only an inch worth of difference, yet it was still outside of the sparrow's narrow range.

The particular response of a borderline patient in terms of the withdrawing or rewarding affect units is evoked, or elicited, much more than it is thought out or elaborated. It possesses a driven or instinctual quality in an interpersonal situation in which this quality is not expected and cannot be readily or easily dealt with.

Fusional attachments and their implications

Fusional attachment is one based on merger—"a joined relationship between the self and the object representations in the internal object world" (Swenson, in Fine, 1989, p. 368). As will be recalled, these part self and part object representations are either positive (the good me/good other), or negative (the bad me/bad other), and different combinations of them are possible.

The nature of fusional attachment varies according to the nature of personality organization. Thus, fusional attachments are more mature and more benign at higher levels of organization (neurotic, normal), and less mature on the borderline level, with the most significant problems in affective and self-other differentiation occurring on the psychotic level.

Much of the early personality development entails what are de facto fusional attachments although different theorists use their own characteristic terms. Fusional attachments are also present in adults with certain types of relational pathology. We are introducing this concept here, because it summarizes complex constellations of affect and relatedness (Swenson, in Fine, 1989, pp. 367–76). It enables us to subsume complex scenarios under a single term which is a great advantage.

The patients with borderline organization show particular characteristics in fusional attachments.

When fusion of positive elements occurs (the good me/good other), then a sense of blissful union will result. On the other hand, when fusion of negative elements occurs, (the bad me/bad other) "affects of fear, rage and persecution" will be triggered (Swenson, in Fine, 1989, p. 369). In a negative fusion "a demanding, deprived self-representation can be fused with a persecutory part-object representation" (p. 370).

The term fusional in this context signifies that the affect and experience of self are embedded within the experience of another in a particular way which recalls the idea of two entities which in some respects function as a single system. For example, conjoined ("Siamese") twins are two entities that may use the same circulatory system or kidney regulation. Siamese twins both are and are not separate entities. In this case, it is affective regulation which is shared.

When positive fusion predominates, the experience of self as whole and worthwhile will be inextricably linked with experiencing the other person as benevolent, protective and idealizable. This, in turn, implies that the experience of self as worthwhile will be dependent on the presence of someone who is benevolent, idealizable or who could be induced by the needy person to have such a role or meaning. The negative fusion, on the other hand, implies that feelings of being deprived will promptly and automatically elicit the sense of another as hostile, depriving or threatening.

The framework of affect and relatedness in a person with borderline features is largely defined by the predictable alterations of positive or negative fusion and their powerful affects.

The particular affective link between feeling needy/deprived and experiencing the other person as hostile and depriving (which occurs as a result of negative fusion) is especially disturbing. It represents a complex constellation of experience of self and others which has several implications.

The affects involved are very intense. In addition, the experience of neediness is complicated by the experience of threat so that the person becomes frightened of his own needs (although he/she can seldom articulate this fear). This complex blend of feelings makes personal involvement with others difficult, both for the patient and for those with whom he interacts.

A borderline patient does not just feel bad, he translates the other person's lack of response or rejection as inevitably signaling either catastrophic abandonment, or if not abandonment, than an expectation that the other person will fulfill his needs in a manipulative way. Thus, when operating under the impact of negative fusion, feeling bad is greatly intensified and elaborated in a paranoid direction, or, equally likely, in the direction of abject helplessness.

This particular blending of affects is a complicated and developmentally more archaic experience than responding in terms of more neutral and less intense affects. It is by no means an inevitable response to social rejection or indifference, or a lack of response on the part of another person.

It is important to point out that the patient does not intend to feel this way. He or she is experiencing something which is not intended.

In the context of borderline affective experience, the sense of another as a hostile, manipulating or somehow threatening presence is not (or not primarily) the result of a cognitive distortion as is the case in paranoid disorders. It is not a well-defined sense of danger which is triggered by a delusion that someone specific is intent on harming him in some specific way (Swenson, in Fine, 1989, p. 370). Rather, it is a more pervasive sense of threat which is linked with helplessness and neediness. This experience is closer to the affective experience in childhood when a sense of massive threat could be very readily mobilized, even in response to minor provocation, because the child did not have any means of knowing (due to a lack of experience, not paranoia) whether the mother's lack of response reflected momentary indifference or permanent desertion. Borderline states may thus represent a momentary (albeit intense) regression to an earlier phase.

The troubling affects of the borderline are thus triggered or evoked, not in response to a cognitive distortion, but, rather, in response to a deficit in one important aspect of emotional adaptation—namely a capacity to grasp on an emotional level that hunger is only temporary.

In sharp contrast to the frightening affects of the negative fusion, the positive fusion generates affects of safety and containment by benign and nurturing others. It can evoke a sense of great confidence and elation and it has a quality of expansiveness which is very compelling. The positive fusion has the capacity to evoke the sense of safety or even elation in an almost automatic way. It represents an effortless adjustment of the sense of well-being and for this reason it is very powerful.

The need for positive fusion is not a simple need for social relatedness, but for a relatedness with a particular feeling tone—it is somewhat in the nature of craving. Such a state is sought out not only because it is intrinsically appealing and reassuring, but also because it provides a way of escaping from being trapped in a negative fusion and its accompanying affects of panic and danger. It creates prompt relief from a sense of great vulnerability and enables a person to reconstitute very rapidly.

The relatedness pattern of a borderline individual is thus characterized by powerful constellations of positive and negative fusion which are evoked rapidly and almost automatically in a toggle-like fashion. The patient has very little flexibility and control over these experiences. He is just as powerfully drawn to seek the expansive affects associated with positive fusion, as he is intensely frightened by the threatening affects of negative fusion. When faced with close involvement he (or she) is, in a sense, both phobic and addicted. We might describe this as a pattern of traumatic dependence.

The above pattern of affective extremes is known as "splitting". Object-relations theorists use this term to describe the character of relatedness which exists in terms of powerful yet opposed affective constellations. As discussed earlier, these extremes remain a lasting feature of interpersonal relationships for those individuals whose attachment history did not yield sufficiently those experiences which make possible the development of modulation and integration—a neutral ground.

Internal structure and the nature of object-relations development

The concept of internal structure figured prominently in the preceding discussions of object-relations development. It is typically defined as an "internal representation of an important relationship". The phrase "internal representation" conveys to some extent the idea of a "blueprint" which is an important aspect of its role.

The chief significance of a psychic structure lies in its capacity to organize affect and relatedness. It can be compared to a riverbed which determines the direction of the flow of water. It can also be compared to the weight-bearing structures of a building. These are structures which absorb the impact of physical stress and prevent the house from collapsing.

A change in the psychic structure means that *affect and relatedness will now have to be organized in some qualitatively different* way. Affective and personality development entails such changes. Therapeutic interventions entail very similar changes. Because a qualitative change requires reorganization or replacing of an existing structure, it is often quite disruptive. For that reason, affective development and the development of identity are not smooth and effortless.

In intervening therapeutically on behalf of borderline individuals, one is confronting not so much a lack of a particular skill but rather a faulty weight-bearing structure.

In reviewing the concepts of various object-relations theorists, one is struck with the complexity of their accounts of early development. In these accounts it is impossible to separate the development of affect from the development of identity and relatedness. These three lines of development are mutually entrained. We might characterize their description of early development as *investiture of identity through affect and attachment*.

This intuitive understanding of their mutual linkage and dependence is one of the most worthwhile contributions of object-relations theorists. It has significant implications for our understanding of early development, as well as forms of psychopathology which represent regression to those earlier levels.

The object-relations approach conveys an appreciation (albeit an implicit one) for the fact that affect, for example, is not a single entity but many.

In trying to conceptualize the development of affect and relatedness, it is probably best not to think of a single line or a straight line, but of an evolving landscape or an ecosystem. In a somewhat unexpected way, it is helpful to think of affective development as evolving in a way reading evolves.

Reading is a complex achievement. It too has a prolonged and gradual development with different building blocks or components established at different stages. What a child of four can grasp is qualitatively different from a child at the age of six or eight. Qualitative changes occur leading to eventual mastery and even excellence. We become aware of these changes, but cannot specify when exactly they began. These qualitative changes can be fostered but not forced.

Reading itself is not one thing. While frequently referred to as a skill, it is certainly not only one skill—it reflects an underlying development of a whole range of diverse cognitive and language functions which support it. It is a process whereby we become capable of greater and greater assimilation of the world around us. We also assimilate the world through feelings.

Phenomenology and psychodynamics of borderline experience

The preceding discussion identified several important concepts and mechanisms pertaining to affect and relatedness including fusional attachments, the need for affective containment through other people, and the compelling nature of affective states. These ideas are cornerstones of our approach to the important clinical issues encountered in treating borderline regressions.

The goal of the following section is to integrate some of the key ideas presented earlier with inferences based on my own therapeutic work with pseudoseizure patients.

Borderline patients, or traumatized individuals in the state of borderline regression, experience affective states which have several important features. To begin with, they represent regressed forms of affect. This means that they are qualitatively different from the individual's normal state and are not merely variants of the normal state.

These affective states have been described in many ways. To the extent that it is possible to summarize them, they can be referred to as complex blends of anger and neediness. Complexity is related to the fact that neither borderline anger nor borderline neediness are straightforward psychologically. As will be apparent from the discussion which follows, borderline anger is significantly complicated by neediness and borderline neediness by anger.

While there is no single concept or mechanism which can capture all of the aspects of borderline affective experience, I shall single out one important component to which I have applied the term *"borderline panic states"* as panic is one of the chief components.

Borderline panic states present a therapeutic challenge, both in their own right, and also because they carry a danger of self-destructive acting out. In approaching this complex, but not uncommon therapeutic problem, it is helpful to try and understand in what way is this state different from others and why it merits special consideration.

Based on my own observations, derived from therapy, I would isolate several features which struck me as distinctive.

The distinction between feelings and drives
The regressed affective states are customarily described in terms of "feelings", typically "unmodulated feelings". One of the characteristic difficulties of borderline patients is that they "cannot control their feelings", and one of the common therapeutic goals (whether explicit or implicit) is to help the patient establish the difference between feelings and actions. This goal reflects a very legitimate and often pressing therapeutic concern.

This line of thought is quite understandable and reasonable, yet there is a great deal more to borderline affect than feelings.

In dealing with this problem, it is helpful to recall the traditional distinction between drives and feelings. This is an important theoretical distinction in psychodynamic theory which is, as a rule, forgotten when describing adults, because it is assumed that all adults have only feelings, whereas drives are reserved primarily for sexuality, thirst and hunger. While nearly anyone dealing with affective/ personality development readily acknowledges that there are definite developmental qualitative changes in the nature of affect (regardless of what specific terms are used to describe them), one rarely finds this term applied to the affect of borderline patients. The term "unmodulated affect" does not really capture the driven quality of the panic states.

While borderline patients may experience higher (modulated) forms of affect when they are well, their panic states have a quality of drive. There are several ways in which "feelings" differ from drives. What we normally have in mind when we say "feelings" are integrated forms of affect which have evolved from earlier forms of affective experience, over long periods of social development, and in the context of attachment. They are an outcome of growth, not is first stage. Feelings may possess a wide range of intensity, but somehow, especially in this culture, they are defined as something which an individual is capable of controlling. Indeed, this capacity to control one's feelings is seen as one of the key features which define an adult personality.

In addition to qualities of modulation and control, feelings also have content. Typically, we think of feelings as being about something or about someone or for someone. People who express their feelings in the right way are said to have good form. Content or form implies that the feelings are appropriate to the social environment in which they take place, that they are relevant and congruent, as a result of which the individual is somehow in accord with others. This is unquestionably a desirable goal of social development, and society could not function with any degree of stability and comfort if its members could not eventually acquire such forms of affective expression.

In borderline regressed states, the affect differs markedly from the above description. The regressive change takes place along several important dimensions. Characteristically, the affect becomes more intense and can rapidly deteriorate. Borderline panic states are typically thought of as being triggered by a fear of abandonment. While this is certainly one of the key issues, the affect itself need not be so specific. It readily regresses into an amorphous state which is simultaneously *very diffuse and very intense, yet may not be about anything in particular* (resembling a signal which has high urgency and low resolution).

This combination is often very unpleasant and threatening. The lack of content—a state which is about *nothing in particular*—is very disturbing in and of itself, since affect is normally attached to something, if not a person, then a problem, or a goal, or even an idea. The lack of content adds an element of confusion to the sense of depletion.

This state of depletion and confusion is not merely a negative feeling; it involves something much more fundamentally wrong. It can be compared to an abraded landscape or an abraded surface, a *lesioned state*. The patient may be facing (albeit sometimes briefly) a vacuum.

To the extent that the above experience can be characterized better, the fear of abandonment, especially catastrophic abandonment, is often an important component of the picture, although this does not mean that the patient can acknowledge it, or even recognize it as such.

The patient's affective state could be described as a blend of anger and hunger. He (or she) is not really experiencing feelings, but a driven state which he is seeking to rectify promptly, immediately and without being made aware of his need (as is consistent with fusional attachments). The patient's chief psychological goal in this state is not to verbalize it or control it, anymore than a person who is hungry is interested in symbolizing or controlling hunger. The borderline patient is behaving as if hungry. But unlike a hungry person who has a simple goal, the hungry borderline does not have a clear goal, only an intense drive to be made better.

Internal assault and affective silence

The patient is filled with a sense of traumatic lack—a *"great inconceivable hunger"*. I have adopted this term from en essay about Thomas Bernhard, a famous Austrian author (in the original "ein grosser, unergreiflicher Hunger"; the author of the essay is unfortunately unknown).

As intense as this state is, however, it is an inarticulate hunger in response to which the person feels both driven and helpless. Unlike biological drive states which organize behavior in pursuit of a clear goal, this particular state does not permit the patient to resolve it in any simple way. A sense of traumatic lack may be experienced as hunger, but it can easily spill over into anger or an alarming sense of helplessness or, very often, all three together.

Unformulated experience

Borderline regressed/panic states can be viewed as "unformulated experience". This is a term borrowed from hermeneutics (Stern, 1997). We might define unformulated experience as something which is not yet an idea, or not yet a memory .The "unformulated" experience is a much more accurate term than "unmodulated", because it stresses the fact that the patient does not initially understand what he or she is confronting. He is driven to reduce a drive state yet does not know what the drive is about. The experience has not yet been processed or even named. While this processing may occur rapidly, if someone helps the patient by establishing the correct empathic link, while it lasts, the panic state appears unknowable.

Dealing with unformulated material—points of technique

How to approach the patient who is struggling with unformulated material?

You are searching for something. Are you able to tell me what you need?

If the patient cannot formulate the answer, or gives a vague answer which reflects chiefly frustration and confusion, the following statement may help.

Whether you can tell me or not, I will remain here and we will try to understand it together.

These two statements communicate to the patient several important points: (a) that the therapist understands that the patient is searching for something; (b) that he/she (the patient) may not be able to define what he is seeking or even experiencing; (c) that not being able to define one's experience is a legitimate position and (d) that therapy will go on regardless of the patient's confusion and immobilization.

Are you trying to hold on or get rid of?

This statement may appear very abstract, but actually deals with the patient's confusion and his/her fear of disorganization. Borderline panic states have a centrifugal quality—the patient may feel as though exploding from within. The self is experienced, not as a center of calm, not as a focus, or firm ground, but as a launch pad. Under normal circumstances, the self is experienced as a force which gathers things into oneself, which organizes and stabilizes. By contrast, in borderline panic states, the self is experienced as a source of chaos, as a vortex from which things fall apart.

This question concerning attempts to hold onto or get rid of something speaks directly to the fundamental aspect of orientation—the difference between the inside and the outside of ourselves. This difference has to do with the difference between oneself and the outer world. This crucial distinction is lost in a traumatic way in a disorganized state. The above statement is in a way a verbal equivalent of pressing one's hand against a wall repeatedly. In doing so, one heightens the reassuring sense of difference between oneself and the outer world. It is an effort to recover orientation.

Are you trying to feel or not to feel?

This question deals with a similar issue. It is an attempt to: (a) acknowledge the patient's confusion and communicate that it is acceptable to be confused; (b) to help define the patient's struggle against contentless yet overwhelming affect; and (c) it acknowledges the therapist's understanding that the patient is not dealing with a clearly defined issue, or one specific feeling as opposed to another specific feeling, but with a mass of affect which threatens to traumatize him and which he is trying to escape.

An equivalent statement might be:

Can you tell me what you are feeling or does it just hurt?

This question also communicates an appreciation of the patient's fear of being traumatized by his own affect—affect which he/she may not even be able to identify.

Loss of demarcation in panic states

While panic/regressed states may have an abrupt and intrusive beginning, they are also very fluid. Once they begin, the experience may be closer to the feeling of being flooded than to confronting some well-defined outside obstacle or threat. Experience which lacks demarcation points (excluding, of course, oceanic and euphoric/ecstatic states) can be very threatening. Individuals who are struggling with such states may try to provoke strong affect in others in order to create provisional markers which they lack.

In this situation, the patient is asked to make a conscious effort—not to control the feeling—but to simply report to the therapist as soon as they become aware of the feeling emerging, and later to report when the feeling begins to fade. Focusing on the beginning and the end, i.e. on the end points of an experiential state, assists in defining the state a little better. As in land surveying, the end points are the beginning of a rudimentary definition.

The challenge of mapping silence
The above phrase captures to some extent the therapist's task (as described in the preceding discussion) of helping borderlines in the midst of their panic states to deal with a great intensity arising from within which has no name, no memory and no anchor in the outside world. It is less of an internal signal, less of a feeling than an internal assault, i.e. affect which is experienced as both intrusive and assaultive.

Anger and acting out are provisional external anchors which feed back to the person a sort of a definition, but at a great cost and without permanent benefit.

As odd as it may sound, borderlines who are frequently assumed to be most dramatic of clinical conditions are actually characterized by a sort of silence, *affective silence* in the midst of great intensity and urgency—a terrain without demarcations. Dealing with their panic states is looking for an area of definition, of contrast—helping to create a territory. To create a territory means to intervene therapeutically against their experience of terror retrogressions and loss of home.

The role of projective identification
Projective identification is one of the chief defenses employed by borderline individuals. However, it is also found in traumatized individuals, for example, in pseudoseizure patients who have regressed traumatically.

The chief aim of projective identification is to deal with states of depletion/confusion/anger and to avert the danger of further panic and disorganization. In this particular defense, the patient deals with threatening affects by evoking them in another person. Thus, if the patient feels intensely angry and helpless, he will elicit those feelings in the therapist. The patient is not aware of this mechanism; nor is this mechanism based on a conscious hostile intent. It is a very powerful defense which stems from an early stage of affect maturation when the child could not deal with strong affects and frustrations except through another person who would make them less threatening through empathy and continuity of connection (recall earlier discussion of Bion). With maturation, the nature of affect and relatedness changes, and the child gradually acquires a capacity to tolerate and neutralize threatening affect by himself. This does not imply that he does not rely on others to make him feel better, however, he does not rely on projective identification in a compulsive or a pervasive way.

The relief provided by eliciting the threatening affect in others occurs in an automatic way—it is not a reasoned strategy. The automatic quality of this defense makes it very powerful. A powerful mechanism of this kind is essential in early stages of development to protect the child who is helpless.

If such a mechanism is used by an adult, however, especially if used pervasively, it can be very destructive as it recreates, on a routine basis, intense and unpleasant affect in others, as well as a sense of helplessness—in a way, it immobilizes the other person. The person who is the target of this defense, paradoxically, does not understand why they are, abruptly and unexpectedly, experiencing anger or helplessness. The patient, as well, only feels assailed by vague but intense inner threats which he (or she) is urgently seeking to escape. This is a particularly challenging aspect of projective identification.

The ultimate aim of projective identification is to elicit a response in another person that will somehow detoxify the intolerable affect and help the patient feel less alarmed. This aim, however, is not always apparent. If this reassuring response or feedback is not forthcoming, further attempts to provoke the person into action through anger are likely which achieves the opposite effect from the one intended, and the behavior may deteriorate.

The patient feels driven to coerce the other person to provide affective containment. As intense as those efforts might be, the patient cannot ask for nurturance directly. This is because he can only experience the awareness of his need and his dependence on another person in a traumatic way. For this reason, he resists being made aware of his need, and is likely to respond with shame or rage if he is made aware of it. The aim of projective identification is to protect the patient from experiencing his neediness directly.

Points of technique

Dealing with projective identification is not a simple task—indeed it is probably one of the most challenging issues in psychotherapeutic management. The therapeutic technique cannot be condensed into a single set of guidelines. However, in the following section, we shall attempt to establish a set of guidelines which is organized around some issues which figure prominently in this clinical situation.

Dealing with projective identification is not a single response. The therapeutic intervention is best conceptualized as a therapeutic approach or process which consists of several components or phases. To begin with, the therapist needs to deal with intense negative affects which the patient "deposited" in them. These affects are typically evoked very unexpectedly, and may or may not reflect the general tone of the material which is being discussed. Thus, the patient may find some particular issue exquisitely painful and promptly regress, yet respond to a much more serious issue without difficulty. Consequently, the issue which causes regression may, from the standpoint of the therapist, be quite unpredictable.

For all these reasons, recognizing that the projective identification is taking place is very difficult since the material which the patient provides is often very impoverished and very stereotypic. At such a time, the patient shows minimal interest in understanding or verbalizing what he/she feels, or indeed doing anything much with it. Instead, this communication is replaced by anger. The anger may be intense and have an air of conviction about it, although it often does not make sense to the therapist. The patient may also accuse the therapist of being angry.

At this juncture, an impasse can easily occur, because the patient appears as though he cannot be moved from his state. The empathic bridge seems gone.

At this point, it is important to reestablish the empathic connection and reestablishing it is the primary intervention. In order for the empathic connection to be rebuilt, it is first necessary for the therapist to deal with the unexpected negative affects and a sense of immobilization which the patient evoked. Tolerating and eventually diffusing those affects is an important intervention in its own right. If, in spite of the negative affects, the therapist maintains neutrality and does not reject the patient or lose interest in him/her, he has already achieved a great deal to recapture therapeutic ground.

It is very natural for the therapist who has established a good working relationship with the patient and has seen his/her other interventions work, to feel pressured to find the right words and to find "the perfect intervention" in this situation. This pressure is unnecessary. To begin with, a situation in which projective identification is operating is one in which it is especially difficult to find interventions which work. This is one of the main reasons why this process is so destructive in interpersonal relationships. Also, it is questionable if indeed there is such a thing as *the* perfect intervention, or even a single correct intervention in this therapeutic context. For this reason, the therapist should feel free to deal with the negative affects at the pace which he or she can handle. This is, in and of itself, an important therapeutic achievement.

One of the challenging aspects of projective identification has to do with the fact that the therapist often does not understand what the affect, especially anger, is about, and it may not be until the following session that the patient provides enough relevant material to make sense of it. Thus, it is not at all unusual to be left baffled at the end of a session and need to wait until the next session to achieve a sense of closure.

To be left without a sense of closure at the end of a session is uncomfortable, but it is not a failure. The patient did not bring the relevant material which would help resolve the situation, because this is characteristic of the way projective identification works. It should be pointed out that the stereotyped and impoverished nature of the patient's response may be in sharp contrast to his usual approach to the material and to the therapist at other times. The stereotypy of the response does not reflect a lack of ability, but represents a regression in his experiential state and his capacity to relate.

When faced with abrupt negative affect or a sense if immobilization it is helpful for the therapist to consider that these are (a) precisely the affects which the patient is struggling with and (b) that he or she cannot deal with them in any other way. Thus, the therapist is using his own affect as a guide to what the patient might be feeling. As with any other therapeutic strategy, this one should be treated only as a hypothesis to be tested, or explored, not as a certainty.

The possibility of projective identification might be signaled by the presence of affect which is intense, negative, abruptly evoked and evoked without any clear cause. Exploring this possibility might in itself provide a structure in a difficult situation and help build a bridge.

Anger evoked in this context has a special meaning of coercing the other person into providing affective containment from threatening affects and reestablishing a sense of fundamental security for the patient. This is a paradoxical way of achieving a sense of security and accepting someone's anger or negative affect in this particular light is not simple. It is very counterintuitive, and it requires a great deal of flexibility and a very generous empathic stance. The therapist's task is made more difficult if the patient insists (as is often the case) that the therapist is the one who is angry and seems insistent on proving it, without any identifiable objective.

Helping the patient discover and acknowledge his feelings as his own is one of the most well-established therapeutic goals. Dealing with anger is a common focus of psychodynamic treatment. However, anger has many different meanings and is handled by different psychological mechanisms in different clinical conditions. This, in turn, implies that different therapeutic interventions are called for, depending on the nature of anger in a particular case. For example, uncovering repressed or rationalized anger in a depressed individual may have a very different course and may require a very different approach then dealing with anger in borderline regressions or in projective identification. In the former case, a depressed patient may find the discovery that he was angry a liberating experience, and may welcome the opportunity to be finally free of that particular burden. He has (potentially) a sense of mastery over his own anger. He will be able to benefit from the therapist' s interpretation that he might be angry.

A borderline patient, on the other hand, will simply feel *injured* if attention is called to his anger, and will respond with a sense of helplessness, or with more anger. He in no way feels in charge of his anger.

The therapist's approach to handling anger in the setting of projective identification is thus different than in other settings. Anger is not only not repressed, it is manifestly there, yet the patient cannot take ownership of it. He has regressed to a developmental stage of experience at which this is not possible. The therapist thus cannot induce him to do so.

In describing the particular character of anger in projective identification, Kohut pointed out that the patient's communication that the therapist is angry should be interpreted by the therapist as if the patient were saying, "there is anger in the air". This statement does not attribute anger to anyone, yet acknowledges its presence.

If the patient's anger is interpreted in this way, the induced negative affect is much easier to handle, and it is also closer to the patient's actual experience. The patient does not see himself as the author, but as a victim of his own anger, and needs help with it in a way in which a person whose house is on fire needs help from his neighbor. He expects this help in a self-evident way, and receiving help does not carry any implications that he set his own house on fire.

Reconceptualizing or "recoding" the patient's anger in this way creates a therapeutic space in which the therapist can again mobilize empathic resources. Why does that matter? Because the need for projective identification implies that the patient has either not mastered an important developmental passage which resulted in the capacity to contain affect, or has regressed temporarily because of trauma.

Object-relations clinicians would argue that an empathic response in this crisis does much more than provide temporary relief. They see empathy as a mechanism of structure building. During critical developmental stages in childhood, modulation of affect and capacity to contain powerful affects are achieved through the cumulative impact of many small instances of tolerance and empathy (rather than one special event). In regressed states, an empathic response likewise helps the patient develop a greater capacity to diffuse overwhelming affects. This implies that providing someone with a background of tolerance and empathy is in a sense providing materials for a house which shelters them. It is not just offering them a shelter, but helping them build their own shelter.

There is an additional aspect of empathic containment which is noteworthy. In responding to the patient's anger with a neutral/therapeutic stance, the therapist can help neutralize the patient' s fear that his anger will necessarily provoke a punitive or hostile response in the other person. As was noted earlier, this fear is a crucial aspect of the borderline affective dynamics according to which the other person is experienced in highly stereotypic ways: either as a benevolent and protective presence or, if not that, then as *necessarily* a punitive one. Consequently, if the patient cannot elicit nurturance, he or she automatically fears hostility—not as a possibility—but as an inevitable and inescapable certainty. This fear is a very powerful driving force behind a great deal of urgency which often accompanies personal involvements of patients with borderline regression features. While this fear is not a result of a delusion, it is nonetheless very powerful, and can be quite disruptive, as it creates a sense that one is hopelessly trapped in intense and difficult transactions without any neutral ground.

A therapeutic response in this context helps desensitize the patient with respect to the involvement with other people which he or she experiences as inevitably intense and dangerous. It helps create neutral ground which enables the patient to eventually break out of the extreme and automatic patterns of negative fusion and replace them with responding to others in less poignant and less consuming ways.

If the therapist is reasonably steady in face of the patient's intense and threatening affects, the patient actually learns how to experience more graded and moderate forms of affect. Empathy in this context serves as a mechanism for desensitization or neutralization of extreme affect. Being benign in this situation is a therapeutic intervention. While it is difficult to explain how this process works, it appears that the patient may, given sufficient time and sufficient number of positive experiences of this kind, eventually internalize more mature and easier forms of affect.

A series of such beneficial learning experiences can eventually serve to build a bridge between affective extremes, an intervening area. The realm of modulated affect and neutrality is a realm of psychological safety and internal control. Being able to develop such an area implies that the patient is no longer driven to invest relationships with others with such dramatic meanings and such intensity as if he were fighting for survival.

Neutrality and the therapeutic approach

One of the challenges in developing a therapeutic approach to the patients with borderline regressions has to do with their difficulty in accepting what the therapist says as neutral, as opposed to injurious. There is a strong affective predisposition to perceive what is said as injurious. For the patient, the affective value of even simple statements changes in regressed states. Furthermore, it changes unpredictably. This presents a difficulty, because the situation has not changed (at least not obviously) for the observer, only for the patient.

This is perhaps comparable to the situation in which two people are sunbathing and one experiences sunburn, whereas the other one does not. The sunburnt skin is now hypersensitive and vulnerable which it is not under normal circumstances, and ordinary actions such as shaking hands may present an ordeal for a sunburned person which they certainly do not represent otherwise. Regression, in a way, resembles or feels like traumatic sunburn except that, in a regressed state, the sunburn is not readily visible. The underlying vulnerability typically becomes apparent—not verbally—but through the patient's negative reactions or a sense of frustration.

The approach to an angry/helpless borderline might be summarized as *empathizing with his anger and helplessness, not challenging* him for experiencing them. This does not imply that a borderline individual should never be challenged. He or she should be challenged when therapeutically indicated.

We might recall our earlier comparison to a person whose house is on fire and who expects help with putting out the fire. Anger and/or helplessness are not conceptualized here as something blameworthy which the patient is required to take care of, but as a genuine predicament, not unlike a fire which both he and the therapist join in putting out—a shared task. The idea of a shared task may be communicated by stating:

- We are facing something here which is bad, (or difficult, or scary), or
- Something is happening here which is scary (difficult, etc.)

These phrases communicate to the patient: You have a legitimate problem which we are both responsible for handling. This idea may seem self-evident and applicable to almost any problem in psychotherapy. However, anger and great neediness are affective states which the patient cannot easily own. In particular, individuals in borderline regressions are vulnerable to a sense of shame. Approaching those affects which they are potentially ashamed of as legitimate problems and a shared responsibility creates a non-threatening framework for the patient. It defines the therapeutic situation as one which resembles two soldiers in a foxhole.

At this particular juncture, it is more important that both the patient and the therapist are mobilized in addressing what the patient perceives as threatening, and only later, when the patient has stabilized enough, to explore how the patient might begin to take ownership of his anger.

Saying "*we* are facing something now" instead of "*you* are experiencing something" is yet another way of therapeutically compensating for a developmental deficit or an unfinished developmental task. It is legitimate to receive help if one's house is on fire or if one is struggling across the river on a narrow bridge.

Other meanings of anger—rehearsing the self

Anger in borderline panic states may, in certain individuals, (or at certain times) be a way of "jumpstarting the self". The person may feel as though they will dissolve into nothing if they are not angry. The fact that the anger may not necessarily be about something makes it even more difficult for the individual.

The therapist may explore this possibility by asking:

- Can you get yourself going without being angry?

OR

- Do you sometimes feel that being angry is the only way you can get yourself going?

As I have suggested earlier, individuals in borderline regressions are not "feeling badly". They are feeling empty and/or they are feeling driven to act, without knowing the goal. There is a great deal of difference between those two types of affective experiences. They are not differences in degree, but in kind. Having specific feelings about a specific issue, or a specific person or a situation is like a clear signal which means one thing—as opposed to another. Panic states are not a clear signal. In a paradoxical way, as intense as they are, they are also flat. They are states of low closure and low information value.

Additional features of borderline affective dynamics

There is an aspect of borderline affective processing which is of note. This has to do with the need to get rid of affective threat in one fell swoop instead of by gradually working through it. We observed that affective range in this group of patients tends towards extremes with very little middle ground. Middle ground consists of modulated affect and affect which is much more integrated with ideas. Such affect can be expressed in words and can, to some extent, be controlled through words.

The borderline individual fears that his/her capacity to establish this kind of middle ground is very fragile, and that, once achieved, he/she could not hold it. He does not really trust himself to hold onto symbolizable and verbalizable affect, and he fears that he cannot hold onto people who matter to him in such a way. It is not just that he cannot achieve modulated affect—he does not trust it in the first place. He needs to be convinced emotionally that there is safety in modulated affect and mature relationships.

A person with such affect dynamics operates emotionally against the background of fear that he cannot rely on himself to ensure that his needs will be met with any degree of consistency. There is a strong reliance on and craving for positive fusion in which needs are fulfilled in an *automatic* and *inspirational way* (*i.e. charismatically*). Likewise, with affective threats or fears, he does not trust himself to work through an affective threat on his own. He feels much more secure if he is able to eliminate troublesome emotional states in one feel swoop. This by no means implies some form of "emotional laziness", because he certainly does not spare himself powerful and demanding affects.

An individual who is trapped in this dilemma operates as if he were profoundly convinced that if he cannot be rid of an internal threat in a one-step process, he will be promptly and inevitably overwhelmed.

A very important therapeutic goal is to help the patient work with an internal threat in a gradual way until he begins to gain confidence that he will not cave in or break apart if the internal threat is not magically and instantaneously dispelled by someone's charismatic presence. As this developmental process begins to gain momentum, the patient will begin to acquire emotional assurance that affective states of low closure, while not pleasant, are not catastrophes. Not being catastrophes, they can be tolerated well enough to prevent serious acting out or panic.

The affective threat lessens, as the patient learns, so to speak, to distribute its impact with an empathic therapist over a period of time. Meanwhile, he learns to develop affective states which are gradations of discomfort, rather than a single overwhelming experience. Discomfort—but not a catastrophe.

Experiencing discomfort without lapsing "into a catastrophe" is a crucial change in affective growth. It is a qualitative difference. A qualitative difference means considerably more than merely feeling better or feeling less threatened. It means that an individual is now organized on a different level and processes affect in a different way (emergence of structure).

The emergence of affective gradations or an affective range in place of paroxysmal affect is an indication that more mature and manageable affect is being established. Such affect, in turn, provides the patient with a mechanism or with a tool with which he can chip away at an internal threat, instead of craving instant relief.

A note on the capacity for control

As we have noted earlier, control over one's own actions and affective states represents one of the most valuable goals of socialization. In the setting of therapeutic management of patients who have regressed to the level of functioning of borderline syndromes, this issue assumes special significance. As a great deal of human suffering can ensue from various forms of acting out—therapeutic methods which aim to strengthen the patient's capacity for control are of unique value in this context.

Bearing this important goal in mind, a clinician needs to be aware, however, that capacity for control is not a single entity. We have excellent reasons for referring to this function of the personality at times as a single function, much as it is useful to refer to memory or concentration as single functions. However, control is many things.

We all know that children grow in their capacity for control over their actions and affects, and while this growth may at times appear slow, the outcome (barring adverse circumstances) is usually positive. Yet it cannot be said that that growth occurs *because* they exert conscious control.

We tend to attribute control of behavior to what is popularly known as "will power". While control over one's actions certainly appears outwardly as will power, this term obscures, rather than reveals the nature of developmental processes which actually establish control.

Among the many components of this complex (and not fully understood) process, neurological maturity ranks high. It is difficult to imagine how capacity for control could be established without this foundation. Beyond that, what psychological processes might be important?

Secure attachment is of great significance in establishing "internal controls". Internal controls are not just internalized experiences of adults exercising good judgment and control. To an even greater extent, internal controls are embedded in memories of adults with whom the child had a secure attachment. Secure attachments contain and integrate anger and they free the child from a painful urgency to act. This process does not occur in an obvious or explicit way, yet it does occur. Thus, the benign presence of others enables the child to establish a smooth integration of affect and action in which the need to control does not impose itself as an intrusive and urgent goal.

In addition to secure attachment, intellectual development and language are each a powerful medium in which affects can be contained, defined, elaborated and refined.

In approaching control as a clinical question and a therapeutic priority, especially with borderline regressions, it is helpful to understand that one is not dealing solely with a regression in the capacity for control. It might be helpful to adopt a wider and more flexible theoretical approach which views control as a final common pathway of successful adaptation. Conversely, a breakdown in the capacity for control may be caused by any number of different mechanisms.

The successful adaptation which ultimately results in the capacity for control calls for an optimal integration of multiple personality systems, including affect and attachment. This particular view of a capacity for control permits us to mobilize a wider range of therapeutic interventions, some of which act to strengthen a sense of continuity of self and repair a sense of fragmentation. These interventions, in turn, have nothing to do with a capacity for control in a narrow sense.

A note on additional therapeutic modalities

The material presented in this section (as well as the remainder of the book) applies chiefly to outpatient therapy. A pseudoseizure patient who has regressed to the level of functioning characteristic of borderline syndromes may require additional treatment modalities which may include in-patient psychiatric treatment. The work of Glen Gabbard is particularly noteworthy in this regard and the reader is referred to his publication (Gabbard, 1986).

Select contributions from self psychology

Narcissistic vulnerability and other problems of self-cohesion

Fundamental concepts

Self psychology is a school of psychodynamic theory and therapeutic practice which has emerged from the theoretical formulations of Heinz Kohut. In the course of his practice, Kohut encountered patients whose problems could not be adequately addressed by traditional psychoanalytic concepts, for example, conflict. Prominent in the clinical picture of these patients was a "specific vulnerability: their self-esteem is unusually labile, and in particular, they are extremely sensitive to failure, disappointments and slights" (Kohut and Wolf, 1978, p. 413).

He came to believe that, rather than being due to a particular conflict, these problems were attributable to a broader deficiency—"a weakened or defective self"(Kohut and Wolf, 1978, p. 414).

In addition to noting the patient's persistent problems with self-esteem, Kohut also observed that they tended to develop certain characteristic patterns of relating to the therapist (i.e. forms of transference). He noted an intense need to elicit accepting and confirming responses from the therapist, or else to perceive him in an idealized light as a source of strength and calmness with whom they could merge psychologically (p. 413). He called the former process of providing acceptance and confirmation *"mirroring"*, and the latter process of merging with someone else's strength and calmness—*"idealization"*. If the patient's predominant interpersonal style in therapy is to elicit mirroring responses from the therapist, he is said to have developed mirror transference. If, on the other hand, he is responding largely in terms of idealization, he is said to have developed idealizing transference. To these two powerful mechanisms of validation which anchor and stabilize the self, he later added a third one, namely, *alter ego or twinship* transference which refers to seeking individuals with whom one can experience a sense of "essential likeness" (Kohut, 1984, p. 194).

From the patients' intense need to mobilize responses from the therapist which would make them feel more vital and more secure, Kohut eventually concluded that he was dealing with processes which were not limited to therapy, but reflected something much more far-reaching and fundamental about the nature of the development of the self.

In this context, self could be described as "core of personality" (Kohut and Wolf, 1978, p. 414), or as an internal organization or mental structure which imparts stability to the personality and its actions and moods. Its key functions are to provide "cohesion and coherence" and to prevent the personality from fragmentation. On page 414, we read:

> The adult self may thus exist in states of varying degrees of coherence, from cohesion to fragmentation; in states of varying degrees of vitality, from vigor to enfeeblement, in states of varying degrees of functional harmony, from order to chaos. Significant failure to achieve cohesion, vigor or harmony, or a significant loss of these qualities after they had been tentatively established may be said to constitute a state of self disorder.

The self is thus an internal structure which ensures integrity of functioning. Kohut's major contention was that this structure develops in a particular way, namely by an individual being exposed to specific types of nurturant experiences. Those include the experience of mirroring, idealization and twinship. As noted earlier, mirroring involves giving someone acceptance, responding to their gifts, enjoying them (Kohut, 1987, p. 256). It is a powerful tool for making another person feel recognized and significant. It is a signal to the child that others derive pleasure in who he or she is.

Twinship experiences are yet another way of feeling valued—knowing that one's experiences are like other people's, that one is not an outcast or an outsider, or someone bizarrely different. Twinship experience provides the child with a sense of belonging to a fellowship of other people from whom one has a reason to expect acceptance and solace in times of need.

Finally, idealization provides its own avenue of psychological survival through an emotional merger with someone who is experienced as both benign and very powerful. The purpose of idealization is to allow someone who feels very frightened, unsure or threatened to seek refuge in someone else's greatness—before they have the time or resources to work things out for themselves. Idealization is not a reasoned or a logical process. Rather, it is an emotional strategy arising out of a sense of urgency and vulnerability in which another person is endowed with powerful meanings. By idealizing such a person one finds relief and orientation.

Kohut saw the above experiences as not only beneficial, but as essential building blocks without which the self cannot be established in full strength. We might characterize his view of the developmental path as a growth of structure through confirmation of value.

A question arises as to why these so-called self-object experiences are so important in the development of self. They are important because they provide the foundation of motivation and pleasure, as well as energy, from which the child can draw to accomplish what he needs in order to grow. They constitute "grounds of hope" (Thomas Jefferson, 1826).

Mirroring, idealization and twinship experiences are not confined to accomplishing a single developmental goal. They could be aptly described as an emotional venture capital for someone who has not yet developed his or her own resources, or whose resources are so fragile that they could not withstand the many setbacks and frustrations. This is not to minimize the very real cognitive and other adaptive capabilities of the growing child, merely to underscore the fact that affective security is slow to develop. It entails prolonged periods of development during which the individual needs to be, in a sense, emotionally ferried across by others.

Kohut referred to nurturant individuals who make it possible for the child to experience mirroring, twinship and idealization as self-objects and the relationships based on those as self-object relationships. Self-object relationships are thus interactions whereby the child achieves resonance in other people's eyes. They could be described as possessing a charismatic quality which generates pleasure and self-recognition.

Self-object relationships are thus not merely empathic interactions, but interactions which generate specifically a sense of being enhanced and expanded. They are a source of narcissistic supplies. Narcissistic supplies are resources of motivation and pleasure which activate and mobilize the individual.

Kohut felt that feelings are critically important as they help structure and consolidate the self. This implies that the development of internal structure de facto rests on the experience of pleasure, of being evoked in the feelings and memory of another. Such an experience reflects a sense of self-cohesion. Self-cohesion is a direct opposite of and it serves as an affective shield against states of depression, depletion, aimlessness, shame and anger.

Kohut's conceptualized the self as being shaped to a significant degree by particular ways in which the self-object needs for mirroring, idealization and twinship were or were not met in early childhood. If those needs were responded to by empathy and attunement, the self would become strong and resistant to many challenges that are typically encountered—it would have cohesion. On the other hand, if the child's needs were ignored, or were responded to too intensely or inappropriately, the self would lack cohesion and would be vulnerable to fragmentation with associated psychopathology.

Kohut conceptualized the growth of the self as crucially dependent on the child being responded to. "What is responded to and becomes self" (Kohut, 1996, p. 289). A sense of pleasure and self-recognition, which are elicited by a richly responsive environment, provide an affective foundation for a wide range of critically important functions of the personality: a sense of reality, a sense of initiative and a capacity to tolerate delays. It bestows freedom from a painful urgency to act. Thus, a richly responsive environment provides not only an affective foundation for vitality and initiative, but also capacity for control and frustration tolerance.

Kohut considered the ultimate goal of psychological growth as being able to internalize the expanding and enhancing quality of the self-object interactions, to absorb them psychologically—to make them one's own so that they form a part of an internal structure (as opposed to remaining a transient experience). Internalization, in the context of self psychology, refers to a process in which one transforms the nurturant and inspiring experiences which others have provided into one's own emotional reserves. The successful outcome of internalization is an internal structure. In this context, this term refers to a psychological experience of well-being which has been transformed into an asset which permits the person to tolerate the inevitable ups and downs and threats to self-esteem that occur in an average environment.

A capacity to internalize external supports (i.e. to *hold on psychologically* to a sense of well-being) is crucial for the development of a mature personality. Without this ability, the person would only be able to function with massive and continuous external supplies. This stable structure is something we draw upon whenever threatened psychologically by loss, displeasure or disappointment. In a sense, it represents " emotional currency" which backs our investments in the world and allows us to operate in the world.

The internalization of a self-object relationship is fundamentally an internalization of pleasure in oneself. This is not merely a pleasure in a particular achievement (although this is an important part of it), not pleasure as a reward, but a state of pleasure for being who one is, a certain sense of pride of being.

The process of internalization of self-object relationships—i.e. the process of establishing the structure—is not a simple one. It basically implies that something which was once a positive experience (or many) is eventually converted into psychological strength or function of the personality. Self-object function is something which begins as the residue of positive self experiences. It is a kind of memory, but what is most remembered is the mood. It is, in a sense, a mood memory which has become sufficiently stable and consolidated that it is now reliably at the person's disposal.

The growth of this internal structure which ensures a basic psychological tone of well-being and provides a foundation of confidence to face any number of challenges does not take place automatically. It does not take place by unconditional gratification either, but, rather, by "optimal frustration". Those optimal frustrations, are "minor, nontraumatic failures in the responses of the mirroring and the idealized self-objects" which force the individual to become slightly more independent (Kohut and Wolf, 1978, p. 416).

Because these frustrations occur *gradually* (a key feature) and are *not drastic* (also a key feature), they do not evoke abrupt drops in mood and self-esteem and they do not generate intense dysphoria. Rather, they evoke minor displeasure which can be repaired. They could be considered manageable hurdles.

An optimal frustration is thus a teaching tool, as it were, as it permits the individual to face the challenge without being overwhelmed by it. Being exposed to a number of *minor, reparable and transient* self-esteem setbacks allows the individual to consolidate a more permanent foundation of self-esteem. This process whereby the self-soothing function is eventually established in the personality is referred to as "transmuting internalization" (Kohut and Wolf, 1978, p. 416).

In his view of development, Kohut focused specifically on the experiences of mirroring, twinship and idealization which evoke a sense of identity and value in the individual, i.e. experience of self-cohesion. As we noted earlier, self-cohesion is an affective foundation, which supports a wide variety of functions: sense of reality, vitality, initiative, regulation of mood and self-esteem, as well as capacity to tolerate anxiety and experience frustration without having to act out impulsively.

Experiences which foster self-cohesion (mirroring, twinship and idealization) have several characteristics. One of them has to do with the fact that the need for such experiences continues throughout our lifetime. While they are critically important to the growing child to help set down foundations of the self, they are also needed later on, at many points throughout life, to help maintain the self in the state of narcissistic equilibrium. Narcissistic equilibrium is a state in which a person has sufficient emotional supplies to underwrite his goals and functioning in the world. It is the opposite of a sense of compulsive neediness, emptiness and anger.

Kohut conceptualized the need to be responded to (a so called narcissistic or self-object need) as something which continues to be essential to the person, even after the self has been successfully established. The presence of a strong internal structure (similar to energy-producing adenosine triphosphate in the cell) which supplies motivation and pleasure and a capacity for self-soothing and self-control is, of course, a precondition for experiencing narcissistic equilibrium. However, it is not sufficient, by itself, to maintain the equilibrium. It does not imply that person is now forever set anymore than it would be true to say that the need for food, water or air can be met on a single occasion. On the contrary, a person continues to rely on the environment for fresh input and confirmation. Narcissistic equilibrium of the adult is thus not a fixed state or a fixed condition. Rather, it is the result of ongoing transactions with an environment which continues to supply response and validation and in which the individual continues to matter.

Experiences which enhance and support the self in the state of narcissistic equilibrium have another important characteristic, namely, when an individual is significantly deprived of such experiences, he is likely to lapse into a state of narcissistic vulnerability. This state is the opposite of self-cohesion and is characterized by a variety of clinical disturbances, symptomatic as well as characterologic. As will be recalled from our earlier discussion, Kohut maintained that the development of the self was founded in self-object experiences of mirroring, alter ego and idealization. However, he went further conceptually and concluded—based on a wealth of clinical observation- that if a person was consistently deprived of such experiences a variety of psychopathological phenomena would follow. He maintained that the absence of response and validation was harmful and a form of trauma in its own right.

Thus, there are two essential forms of trauma. The first is the classical trauma of death or loss of a loved one or physical/emotional abuse which leave in their wake mourning, conflict and troubled identifications with aggressors or lost loves.

The second kind of trauma stems from indifference. It prevents the person from being soothed, recognized and confirmed in value. Individuals who are traumatized in this way suffer from "sentiments of incompleteness". This is the term used by Pierre Janet—a pioneering French psychiatrist—writing nearly 100 years ago about traits which he observed in some of his patients which would today be considered disturbances of narcissistic equilibrium or narcissistic deficits (Pierre Janet, 1965).

Their experience can be characterized as lacking affective closure. They may engage in maladaptive behaviors in order to elicit feelings and feedback which create an emotional sense of definition.

The nature of the narcissistic bond

In reviewing the nature of self-object or narcissistic needs we emphasized two important features. One had to do with the fact that they continue to be relevant throughout lifetime of an individual—one does not remain in a state of narcissistic equilibrium without ongoing input from others. Mirroring is no less relevant to an older person trying to come to terms with the meaning of his life than it is to a five-year-old who is just meeting life and needs to know that he is worthwhile.

The second characteristic of narcissistic needs is that, although they have to do with feelings, they are much like material supplies, for example, food and water. They have a homeostatic function—which means that they are necessary to ensure balance. Furthermore, they follow cycles of deprivation and fulfillment which implies that a serious or prolonged deprivation will impair the organism's ability to function. Thus, a neutral state does not really exist at the narcissistic level of personality—one has either fulfilled self-object needs or not, just as a person is either thirsty or is not.

The third characteristic of self-object needs has to do with the particular way in which others who fulfill them are perceived by the person. Kohut made an important observation that those who fulfill self-object needs are not experienced as separate individuals, but as extensions of oneself (Kohut 1996).

The person who relates narcissistically expects to exercise the kind of control over self-objects which he or she can only expect to have over his own body or even more, over his own thinking processes (Kohut, 1996, p. 33).

Also, on page 33, Kohut notes:

> The narcissistically fixated individual, in the dimension of his personality with which he relates to others narcissistically, will react to the other person's refusal in the same way we react when our arm does not go up when we want it to go up, or when our words don't come to us, or when we make a slip of the tongue.

He later adds, "we react with a kind of anger, a kind of deep rage, when something which is included in the self is not obeying us"(p. 33).

Frustration of self-object needs does not always lead to anger. Indeed, in a number of instances, it leads to depression, depletion, failures of initiative, or to other pathologic phenomena. However, the intimate connection between a deprivation of narcissistic needs and rage is one of the most intriguing psychodynamic patterns as it is often not readily apparent either to the individuals experiencing it or to others with whom they relate.

The narcissistic bond is thus both very intense and very fragile—there is little room for psychological middle ground. The other person who is identified as a source of supplies is either an idealized benefactor or a villain. The propensity to experience others in this extreme way, and especially, rapid shifts between those extremes, are not due to a lack of intelligence or delusional thinking. Rather, they are directly related to a sense of deep vulnerability and urgency.

This sense of vulnerability and urgency can occur in a variety of psychological circumstances and settings and for a variety of reasons. To begin with, such feelings are easily evoked in young children for very legitimate reasons. Children have no control over their emotional and material supplies and tend to react to nearly all frustration as if it were an emergency. At some level, they fear (without being able to articulate it) that they might be catastrophically abandoned *unless they control others* in an almost *automatic way*. This is why a trivial frustration may be just as likely to trigger a panic-stricken tantrum as a serious threat to their well-being. The emotional distance between being intensely related and connected to a parent, and perceiving them as a witch is short. From the perspective of a child who sees the other in an idealized light as a source of all bounty—as an all-powerful presence—there is no logical reason why this benevolent giant would frustrate them at all unless, of course, they are evil.

An additional reason which adds to the volatile nature of the narcissistic bond is that the needs of a young child are not brief or intermittent. On the contrary, the child has to be surrounded with an entire background of care, not an occasional kind gesture. He cannot, for example, eat on alternate days and have parents available every spring. He also cannot negotiate their presence, and should not be in a position to have to bid for their attention on an open market. He has no choice but to take his parents for granted. In that sense, his mode of relating has a strongly narcissistic foundation which is entirely normal and appropriate until, gradually, he develops social sensitivity and an awareness of other people's viewpoint and other people's needs.

Narcissistic features similar to the ones described above also occur in adults with narcissistic deficits. In that setting, they are again linked to an intense sense of fundamental vulnerability coupled with an urgent need to elicit soothing and mirroring from others—without much negotiation or elaboration. Specific manifestations of these narcissistic vulnerabilities and clinical scenarios in which they play a role will be described in the sections which follow.

The concept of merger

In the context of self psychology, merger can be defined as an experience of emotional union with another person by whose emotional strength one feels nurtured and whose psychological presence and availability are treated as self-evident. One might comment at this point that issues with the role of nurturance are by no means unique to self psychology. Most theoretical and clinical models of human development deal with it in some way. Each of them has a somewhat different emphasis, depending on the nature of clinical problems they are trying to address.

This experience of merger is a psychological state in which one feels emotionally sustained by another person who is not experienced emotionally as anything other than oneself. This is a key characteristic.

We should emphasize that a merger (in the context of self psychology, as well as elsewhere in this book) refers to a quality of feeling—a feeling state—and not behavior.

The experience of merger does not rest on a conscious perception. An individual who is experiencing merger, be it a child or an adult, does not *think* that the other person is physically a part of them. They are not delusional. To say that an individual experiencing merger *perceives* the other person in a particular way, for example, as a part of their own self, is too strong and probably misleading. A child or an adult who is in a state of emotional merger does not perceive anything in a sense of making judgments about the other person. Rather, he *feels* a reassuring sense of continuity with another person in a way that we feel surrounded and permeated with the warmth of a room which we have just entered from the cold—without being aware of the difference between the warmth and our body and without being able to tell where the warmth begins or ends.

Self-object experiences of twinship and idealization are based on merger. They are not negotiated relationships with another person, but, rather, experiences of intrinsic relatedness. The pleasure which stems from this intrinsic relatedness is not something one works for or sets out to achieve as a conscious personal goal. Rather, it is something one becomes aware of or recognizes in an effortless and self-evident way. The spontaneous emergence of the feeling of pleasure in a merger is one of its most compelling features. The person experiencing merger does not wish to articulate how much he is seeking such an experience—he most especially does not want to explain anything to the other person, or, worse, have to work to elicit this sense of smooth emotional continuity. It is the fact that it occurs effortlessly and without any negotiation that makes merger valuable.

Merger is thus an experience of highest emotional quality (although there are exceptions to this rule). Although intensely attractive, it is not easy to manage for several reasons. To begin with, both children and adults experiencing merger (i.e. operating on an essentially narcissistic level) are rarely aware that they are seeking that particular experience. As powerful as the experience might be, a person may not be at all well aware that they are seeking this particular kind of immediate and effortless connection and not some other rewarding interpersonal exchange. Not only are there not really aware of what they are seeking, they are defended against the awareness of the need.

Typically, the awareness of the narcissistic need does not emerge smoothly. It is something one stumbles upon much as one might come up against an obstacle which has no business being there. Its emergence is thus abrupt and disruptive. The ensuing disappointment can be very acute and can rapidly escalate into rage, the reasons for the rage being obscure to both the person experiencing it and the person who disappointed them. In this situation, there is virtually no real transition between the person's normal state and the rage.

The person who is enraged does not really know that he or she expected this kind of smooth emotional connection, this background of nurturance, until the other person shows that they are not "on the same wavelength". The awareness that merger is not forthcoming is like a sudden awareness of the environment turning cold for no reason at all. One experiences it as outrageous, not because one cannot defend oneself from the cold, it is not a question of not being able to take action to bring the warmth back, but because one wanted the sustaining community of warmth—to be surrounded by it and not to be made aware, in an abrupt way, of the difference between oneself and the world. An awareness of difference often carries with it the burden of having to face the world and to negotiate for one's needs and one's place in it.

One of the key characteristics of a merger is the need not to be made aware of the difference between oneself and the nurturing person (self-object)—a need for a state in which one flows emotionally into the domain of someone else's experience, because that is how one feels contained and protected.

A person who is operating emotionally on the level of a merger resists any awareness of a discontinuity between himself and self-object in the same way that the person in the above example resists the sudden disappearance of warmth although he or she can turn the thermostat on in seconds. It is not that the person is helpless in the sense of realistic problem-solving (although this could certainly also be the case). Rather, he desires not to act upon his surroundings, but to be contained within them.

Acting upon one's environment is a very different psychological process from containment. They are two entirely different needs and represent different approaches to relating to one's environment, as well as different developmental levels of adaptation. Obviously, both are needed and each is appropriate for a given life goal or a life stage. For example, one could not build a bridge over a river by emotionally merging with the beauty of the surroundings. On the other hand, one could not experience lasting happiness if, when called upon to appreciate the beauty of the surroundings, for example, on one' s honeymoon, one resisted merging with the beauty of the setting and offered to build a bridge instead.

In discussing the nature of a merger, we have emphasized the need not to be made aware of the difference between oneself and the nurturing presence of another person. It is characteristic of the person who operates on the level of a merger (i.e. narcissistically) that they do not really desire so much the other person, but, rather, or, primarily, their nurturing presence (these are two very different things).

We could call the need to experience a sense of continuity between oneself and the nurturing presence of the other—a need for containment (by another person).

There is an aspect of this need which is noteworthy and requires some elaboration. While very powerful, especially in young children, and also in adults with narcissistic vulnerabilities, as well as in traumatized individuals, this need for containment is paradoxically not really conscious, nor is it easy to make sense of, experientially or conceptually.

The need for containment is similar to hunger and thirst. It is very basic and a significant deprivation sets up states of highly motivated search for fulfillment which, in turn, implies that it cannot be put on hold forever without consequences for a person's functioning.

However, unlike hunger or thirst which are easy to identify as such, the need for containment is not easy to identify as such, because it is so fundamental (much like the need for air). It is a part of our experience of ourselves, yet it is not a part of our vocabulary of the self. It is a form of hunger which is not easy to name. The foundation of the need for containment is a sense of deprivation—a particular form of deprivation which, unlike hunger or thirst, is poorly defined and not really clear either to the person experiencing it, or to the person who could offer the nurturance (unless, of course, they are very empathic and attuned).

It is an experience of lacking something which typically becomes more defined only as the person progresses along the path of being deprived and becomes frustrated or enraged, (or else, disinterested and inhibited). This means that the need for containment frequently becomes manifest in a disruptive and insidious way. In fact, in the setting of narcissistic experience, the sharp, abrupt episodes of rage (or other signs of dysfunctional behavior) are signals that one is deprived. The fact that one typically becomes aware of the need for containment in such a painful and peculiar way is the reason why the narcissistic bond, while very intense and in some ways addictive, is also very easily disrupted and therefore difficult to manage, both for the person who operates predominantly on the narcissistic level and for those to whom they relate.

In characterizing the need for containment as something which is difficult to define and articulate, we should again point out that this difficulty does not stem from any personal deficits. It is not due to intellectual limitations, and it does not imply poor verbal skills (generally). Rather, one is dealing with a difficulty in finding words, or even ideas or images which reflect this particular type of experience.

We could summarize the nature of the narcissistic bond in terms of its two fundamental features. (1) It is a type of relatedness in which a person maintains self-cohesion and self-coherence by means of a merger with an idealized "other", or by a merger with someone who is felt to be, in a very reassuring way, just like oneself. (2) If a merger is not permitted to take place as often and as intensely as the person is driven to seek it, or the merger gets disrupted, a marked tendency to respond with anger (or others signs of dysfunction) becomes very apparent. Thus, a narcissistic bond is not just being significantly driven to seek an effortless connection with others which is natural in and of itself. It is more than longing for a merger. A narcissistic bond is based on a specific dynamic link between the disruption of a merger and anger and/or impairment of functioning.

This particular psychodynamic pattern in which one finds both anger and a persistent need to merge with an idealized self-object is not intuitively obvious. The two components seem to be total opposites. One deals with affiliative needs and nurturance whereas the other deals with aggression.

Kohut's important intuitive discovery was that, at narcissistic levels of relatedness, which characterize early forms of attachment, not only was the boundary line between aggression and attachment tenuous, but he also described clinical consequences of that particular psychological situation.

Narcissistic relatedness and marital relationship

The propensity to form narcissistic bonds has important implications for a person's social functioning. One of the settings in which this impact is most apparent is the family setting, especially marital relationship.

Ikar Kalogjera and his colleagues examined interactional patterns of the narcissistic couple (Kalogjera et al., in Carlson and Sperry, 1998). In their treatment of this complex topic, Kalogjera and his colleagues brought to bear a number of important concepts and themes from self psychology to account for the difficulties which are characteristic of this particular relationship. Their conceptualization of the relationship difficulties in the narcissistic couple emphasizes the following issues:

- The role of idealization, twinship and mirroring
- Anger and withdrawal
- Role of curative fantasy
- Role of traumatic de-idealization

In a narcissistic couple, both partners suffer from significant narcissistic vulnerabilities. This vulnerability can be described as "the increased sensitivity to disappointments and extreme difficulty in dealing with real or imagined rejections, slights and failures" (Kalogjera et al., in Carlson and Sperry, p. 218). It should be pointed out that some degree of narcissistic vulnerability is present in many individuals and can also be found in many relationships. However, it is especially pronounced in the narcissistic couple. For them, the narcissistic vulnerability is not limited to an occasional regression in response to major adverse life events or losses. Rather, there is a more or less permanent background of vulnerability which places the relationship at risk.

Narcissistic vulnerability in the partners stems from adverse childhood experiences, specifically from the failure to receive an adequate amount of such experiences as mirroring, twinship and idealization with calm and reassuring parental figures. This pattern is referred to as "repeated self-object failures". This term is synonymous with Kohut's concept of trauma of nonresponse discussed earlier where an individual is traumatized by indifference in a situation in which the other person's response is vitally needed and a child has reason to expect it (that is to say, where narcissistic supplies provided through mirroring, twinship and idealization are developmentally appropriate and necessary).

A childhood background which is significantly and chronically lacking in reassuring and self-confirming experiences leaves the spouses vulnerable in several ways. They are needy much of the time, and are in search of effortless connections such as those which are present in merger. We might describe a narcissistic couple as one in which spouses are in search of charismatic connection, and the kind of immediate, effortless relatedness which characterizes the narcissistic bond and which does not require that they work for it or even articulate it. They are seeking someone to mirror them, to feel that the spouse is not just a partner, but a soul-mate (twinship), and, especially, they are seeking to unite with the other person's strength and calmness. Thus, they are not looking for an occasional kind gesture or a pat on the back. Rather, they are seeking a steady background of smooth mergers and implicit understanding.

We might point out at this point that this particular aspect of their relationship style is very close to the widely popular and accepted concept of romantic love which is an important component of many relationships. However, what sets narcissistic couples apart are two conditions. First, they have a particularly strong need for mirroring and confirmation which they expect to occur implicitly and they tend to relate through mergers and not in other, less interpersonally demanding ways. Second, that longing for mirroring and merging with others stems largely from a need to repair the damage done to the self during the early years when parents did not provide sufficient opportunity for the child to be mirrored and soothed by the reassuring presence of a calm parent. Thus, in a narcissistic couple, partners rely heavily on the marital relationship to supplement psychological supplies which were inadequate in childhood. This pattern has been conceptualized by Ornstein and Ornstein, (cited in Kalogjera et al., in Carlson and Sperry, 1998, p. 222–3) as *curative fantasy*. They characterized it in the following way:

> Infantile expectations, "to be made up to", to have past hurts undone and old, frustrated wishes fulfilled, are readily activated in marital relationships. Since these infantile expectations are always compounded by guilt and shame, marital transactions frequently have the appearance of a neurotic interaction between a demanding, guilty child, and a frustrating, punitive, or acquiescing parent.

When the spouse fails to provide a background of smooth emotional continuity, there is a tendency to experience narcissistic injury which is, as a rule, promptly translated into anger.

> Narcissistically disordered couples are especially prone to using defensive reactions of blaming, attacking, counterattacking and distancing, in response to narcissistic injuries. However, such reactions are also restorative attempts to elicit an empathic response from the self-object, which also is an enactment of the initial curative fantasy (Kalogjera et al., in Carlson and Sperry, 1998, p. 225).

The above statement underscores both the complexity of narcissistic relatedness and also its paradoxical nature. To begin with, there is a strong link between great (but poorly or ineptly articulated) neediness on the one hand, and anger, distancing and blaming on the other. This implies that spouses who relate narcissistically not only get angry a good deal (or withdrawn which is a softer variant and has the same function), but they also get angry specifically when they are most needy. They are needy in ways which are not only hard for them to articulate, but they are often threatened, angered or ashamed by their own needs for merging.

The great paradox of narcissistic relatedness is this tendency to get angry or chilly when one is needy and even *because* one is needy—to articulate neediness mainly through anger to which a natural response on the part of the partner is to withdraw. The withdrawal of the partner, however, will only lead to alarm, anger and greater narcissistic injury. The person who is narcissistically injured does not desire withdrawal of the partner. Rather, they want the partner to recognize and fulfill their need for connection amidst all the blaming and anger and in spite of all the blaming and anger.

The above pattern represents a peculiar psychological bind. Dealing with this bind is clearly psychologically very challenging and places exceptional demands on the partner(s). The difficulty is compounded by the fact that both partners in a narcissistic couple are likely to have similar narcissistic vulnerabilities and both expect to be nurtured while simultaneously blaming each other (Kalogjera et al., in Carlson and Sperry, 1998, p. 220).

Repeated occurrence of the above situation is likely to place substantial burden on the marital relationship, and eventually lead to a condition which has been described as "traumatic de-idealization".

The concept of traumatic de-idealization was introduced by Jerald Kay in an attempt to deal with psychological stress experienced by medical students in the course of their professionalization (Kay, 1990). This concept can be summarized as a series of traumatic disappointments in the context of a relationship with significant authority figures whom one needs to idealize in order to be sustained emotionally in a situation where one faces sustained pressure and demand. In arriving at an understanding of this complex psychological situation, several components need to be considered: (1) the psychological situation of the medical student; (2) the need for idealizable authority figures; and (3) impact of traumatic disappointment.

A medical student is faced with a situation that demands sustained levels of performance with respect to academic requirements, effective social functioning, as well as interpersonal giving. There is also the added responsibility of being introduced to a profession which enjoys unique prestige and social significance. The intensity and the sustained nature of these demands make for a challenging situation. The status of a trainee also has intrinsic vulnerabilites of its own as it is essentially a right of passage. A right of passage demands more from the student than merely accumulating a good deal of information and mastering a content area; it requires a considerable amount of personal maturation.

The intensity of the process of medical professionalization and the student's role of a novice create a heightened need for narcissistic supplies and support. This means that he will need to be able to see his teachers/authority figures (faculty and house staff) as idealizable. Idealizable does not mean ideal or flawless, but rather possessing a quality of being admirable, inspiring enthusiasm and fostering identification. Identification with an idealizable teacher who is experienced in much the same way emotionally as idealizable parental figures in childhood is a key element in the process of *emotional identification* with one's profession, especially in being proud to take part in it. Another important function of being able to idealize authority figures who are in charge of one's education has to do with the fact that idealization provides a soothing influence which helps the student bridge many difficult and anxiety-provoking situations.

Idealizable figures have a beneficial impact that extends beyond helping the student with specific issues which are a part of the process of learning any occupation. Rather, they create a background of positive influence which can neutralize many individual hardships and protect the student from becoming demoralized or immobilized.

In addition to the need for idealizable guides and mentors, the student also needs to be able to receive confirming responses from them. If this does not occur, and the student in fact faces the opposite situation in which ongoing indifference, mixed with criticism, especially unjust criticism, are the norm, he may experience traumatic de-idealization which is the result of cumulative impact of a series of "brief, albeit painfully intense disappointments" (Kay, 1990, p. 572).

These traumatic disappointments are not "minor student irritations, frustrations and misunderstandings" (p. 572) which are mostly unavoidable. Rather, they are disappointments which strike at the student's self-esteem in a significant way and interfere with his ability to identify with his profession.

Thus, the concept of traumatic de-idealization refers to traumatic disappointment in a setting in which one needs to be able to idealize others, and receive confirming and supportive feedback from them, in order to accomplish some developmental task or function in some significant role.

Kalogjera and his colleagues (in Carlson and Sperry, 1998) applied the concept of traumatic de-idealization to their understanding of the dynamics of the narcissistic couple. They saw a number of important parallels between the narcissistic vulnerability which characterizes the situation of a medical student (as depicted by Kay) and the way in which spouses in a narcissistic couple are both very reliant on and yet potentially very vulnerable with respect to each other.

To begin with, marriage could be readily seen as both a developmental task and a significant ongoing role for each spouse. In a marriage, spouses are social equals, and not authority figures for each other. However, they need to be able to function as idealizable figures for each other in a way which retains the positive parental quality. Being able to idealize a spouse is not restricted to a narcissistic couple; rather it is (as we noted earlier) a component of romantic love. However, the need for a merger with an idealized image is particularly pronounced in narcissistic couples, because it has a specific function of offsetting a painful sense of lack which stems from not receiving sufficient narcissistic supplies in childhood. Most importantly, narcissistically relating couples are especially prone to being promptly narcissistically injured, and reacting with anger or icy withdrawal if the desired response is not evoked in the partner. The cumulative impact of these disappointments is traumatic de-idealization which has as a consequence not only diminished self-esteem and self-feeling in individual partners, but also doubts about the viability and value of the marriage relationship, as well as reduced investment in it (Kalogjera et al., in Carlson and Sperry, 1998).

In the preceding discussion, the concept of traumatic de-idealization was applied to a clinical setting (narcissistic marital relationship), as well as the situation of a medical student. The latter is not a clinical setting although the difficulties described have clinical implications. We might describe the situation of a medical student as a period of intensified normal adult development with heightened needs for narcissistic support and supplies. In a sense, all major phases of emotional/personality development could be conceptualized as periods of heightened narcissistic requirements, i.e. periods when one is especially dependent on support drawn from self-object relationships.

This support is needed in order to (a) keep the individual mobilized, and (b) to absorb anxiety which inevitably arises from repeated confrontations with new or challenging situations. Similarly, we might argue that increased narcissistic supplies are also needed for any complex role which has to be sustained over a period of time and is not transient.

A heightened need for narcissistic supplies during periods of intense development could be compared to an increased rate of metabolism which, in turn, results in a need for larger amounts of nutrients. This implies that an individual entering a new significant phase of life needs more than rudimentary guidance or a few stock phrases of encouragement. He needs an opportunity, regardless of his age, to experience mergers with individuals who are perceived in an idealized light as calm and powerful. He also needs to be able to receive feedback confirming that he is doing well. Thus, he (or she) requires active support.

If this active support is not forthcoming, or is only forthcoming after a long delay, any number of difficulties may arise, ranging from a sense of chronic stress, feelings of demoralization, of being hungry for praise and, finally, abrupt drops in personal effectiveness leading to an erratic course of personal performance. Regardless of the nature of a specific difficulty which may accompany the individual having to "go it alone", the absence of active support as such is liable to be a problem for many people.

We should qualify this statement by pointing out that people vary in the amount of narcissistic support they require. There are individuals who appear to need only minimal narcissistic supplies and who, in fact, prefer a large measure of independence. However, from the standpoint of self psychology, there is no such thing as a free passage through a developmental stage or a major life role. Active input and interest of others are required.

The role of empathy

Empathy is traditionally defined as the capacity to feel what the other person is feeling. It is a bridge which permits us access to the emotional world of another person and things which matter to them.

A classical tool of therapists, it is both a way of understanding the patient, as well as a form of therapeutic response.

> From the moment when man is born it is empathy, the wordless psychological extension of the human environment to the baby which separates him from the inorganic world: from death, from the meaninglessness of racing solar systems, from incomprehensible spaces, and from the ever more incomprehensible vastness of endless time... It is this expansion of the self beyond the limits of the individual which is the barrier to meaninglessness, to pessimistic despair (Kohut, cited in Strozier, 2001, p. 330-1).

This statement reflects Kohut's view of empathy as a developmental force—something which not only enhances development, but actually drives it. An operative force which allows us to become substantial as humans. A child's investiture into humanity.

While empathy is intrinsically a capacity to feel with another and for another, it is more than a feeling. Kohut's understanding of it as a *barrier* to frightening regressions and loss of identity is a very unique insight.

To some extent, empathy has paradoxical nature. It is a feeling, yet also a mechanism of growth which builds structure of the self and self-feeling, "a kindling light" (Poe, 2002 a). Empathy is often perceived as an esoteric component of human interaction—not substantial, yet its impact is to make us psychologically substantial .At first glance—a concept as different from brick-laying as one can imagine—it is in psychological terms exactly that.

Narcissistic foundations of normal relationships

Parent/child, marriage, employee/employer and individual/society can all be characterized as fundamental relationships. We use the term fundamental because these particular relationships anchor the emotional life of the individual. Also, these are relationships through which the life of society is organized and stabilized. It could be argued that all of these relationships have a narcissistic foundation. There are several reasons for this: their intensity, the fact that they span the individual's entire life, a significant power differential among people involved, and the presence of implicit mergers.

The people involved in above relationships share the essential tasks of life. That makes them potentially very intense and even compelling. To say that fundamental relationships have a narcissistic foundation does not imply that they do not also contain a very significant component of realistic, negotiated and task-oriented mode of relating. They clearly do; otherwise, the important life tasks with which they are concerned could not be accomplished. However, insofar as a person cannot really choose to be in them, but feels compelled to join others to form such relationships, they contain a narcissistic element.

The narcissistic element has to do with the essential (not pathological) needs of the individual. This is most obvious in the case of a child who does not join a family, but is born into it, and who clearly needs others for extended periods of time and whose start in life is intimately tied with how and whether they respond to him. The child cannot choose not to need narcissistic supplies, because they make him psychologically buoyant and viable.

The marriage relationship, although socially among equals, is not entirely an egalitarian relationship either, in the psychological sense, because the partners are mutually responsible for fulfilling each other's needs for mirroring and idealization. Also, one partner may be specifically charged with the role of a rescuer or a healer of past wounds. These three functions, particularly idealization and healing past wounds are, by definition, the roles of someone more powerful psychologically. They are the roles of a symbolic if not actual parent.

Work settings contain a strong component of realistic and task-oriented mode of functioning and elaborate structures and hierarchies are built to ensure that particular goals are reached. Work settings determine, in a very powerful way, the livelihood and social identity of the individual who works there. This means that the individual's sense of worth is affected in a very comprehensive way. The work environment provides ongoing opportunities for experiencing both pride (with achievement), as well as shame with a job failure or a job loss. On the one hand, the individual's commitment and investment in work serve as an important source of narcissistic supplies. On the other, the very intensity and force of that commitment are a source of narcissistic threat—if the job is jeopardized, the individual faces a significant narcissistic threat.

The above relationships, when functioning well, provide a background of well-being and psychological constancy and they nurture self-esteem. However, they are easily disrupted. The parent, or employer (to some extent, the spouse as well) has the role of someone who provides narcissistic supplies and resources. Such a person is often experienced as very powerful and in control of all the resources. The psychological danger inherent in this situation is the fear that the resources will be taken away in an abrupt and catastrophic way. Thus, there is very little middle ground. To the extent that the relationship has (or is perceived as having) a strongly asymmetric quality, and the other person is seen as having control over one's entire well-being, the person who is not in a position of power is vulnerable to narcissistic injury.

In addition to their intensity and the fact that they affect the individual for extended periods of time, fundamental relationships share another characteristic. They are organized, in part, on the level of a merger, i.e. a sense of assumed connection with others which is reassuring.

Mergers are not the only way in which fundamental relationships are organized. However, there is a component of the relationship which has the psychological quality of a merger. That is most evident in the relationship between the parent and child. The child must be able to elicit admiration, confirmation and soothing, as well as a sense that he is like other people in order to consolidate a sense of self.

Merger is a significant component of a marriage relationship (or other partnerships) as well, not just in the case of the narcissistic couple, but more generally, since it provides a context for the ongoing satisfaction of needs which relate to self-esteem and a sense of pride and vitality.

Work settings are typically taught of as being socially organized around specific work objectives, and we rarely think of them as a context in which relating on the level of a merger has any role at all. While they are indeed organized, to a large extent, along rational lines which are most suited towards achieving their particular institutional tasks, the social and psychological matrix of work settings is often more complex, and contains other elements as well.

As we have seen in the case of the medical student, there is a need for ongoing feedback and a need for idealizable figures. Thus, there is a need for relevance and for a response whose meaning is not exhausted in a grade or pay—a need analogous to being seen as a "good son" by one's preceptors or supervisors. This and related needs are by no means limited to medical students and other young adults undergoing rigorous and stressful professionalization, but is a much more ubiquitous need.

This need, however, is not always apparent for several reasons. People vary in the extent to which they are aware of their self-object needs. They may also be hesitant to express them, or even ashamed of acknowledging them for fear of being considered immature. Furthermore, self-object needs are not easy to identify. Typically, they are expressed in indirect ways, chiefly through symptoms which appear when they are not met, such as hunger for praise, a sense of chronic imbalance between what one gives and what one gets back, and a drift in personal effectiveness.

The opportunity to rely on benign paternal or maternal figures (without having to launch an exhaustive search for them) is not a prerogative of children or individuals in training who traditionally need mentors. Mergers with benign idealizable figures have an emotional impact which goes well beyond the relationship with a particular individual. Such a merger stands for, in emotional terms, the contact with a wider social world which is presumed to be benign and orderly in the same way that having reassuring and supportive parents creates in the child a sense that the wider world is also benign and safe.

We can thus characterize fundamental relationships—parent/child; marriage; employee/employer and individual/society—as having, in part, a narcissistic foundation. This conclusion rests on the following observations. Fundamental relationships are intensely important, they span large sections of the individual's life, are not really relationships among equals (in the psychological sense), and they contain implicit mergers which ensure a sense of continuity of security and normalcy.

Having a narcissistic foundation, however, renders the fundamental relationships inherently vulnerable to disruption, because the narcissistic bond, albeit intense and compelling, is, by its nature, volatile. One of the ways in which this disruption occurs is through a disruption of implicit mergers in the family, marriage or work relationships. In fact, one may conceptualize trauma as a disruption of mergers which typically stabilize psychological functioning of the individual and which need to be there, at least in a subtle form, and without the individual having to struggle to ensure their presence. Disruption of mergers, in turn, can lead to traumatic disappointment, traumatic de-idealization and regression in functioning.

The preceding discussion dealt, to a large extent, with forms of narcissistic vulnerability which may arise in individuals who operate in unempathic environments where they are faced with prolonged and significant deprivation of narcissistic supplies—the trauma of not being responded to. Thus, Kohut focused on this particular kind of trauma which by itself can create a good deal of psychological disturbance. However, in our view, the concepts of narcissistic vulnerability in general and traumatic de-idealization in particular, can also be applied in the setting of physical or sexual traumatization.

Trauma victims and traumatic de-idealization

The dynamics of physical and sexual traumatization of either children or adults is complex and contains a number of diverse psychological processes and mechanisms (discussed in Section I of this book, as well as in psychoanalytic contributions in Section II). There is a proportion of traumatized individuals, which includes pseudoseizure patients, (particularly chronic cases) for whom the dynamics of traumatic de-idealization is applicable and can help explain some aspects of the clinical picture.

A person who was traumatized, especially if trauma took place in the context of the parent/child or marriage relationship, has, in a sense, two psychological tasks. He or she has to deal with the specific traumatic event and the person who hurt them. In addition, however, there is a need to deal with traumatic disappointment and, eventually traumatic de idealization, if the person who hurt them is someone on whom they are rely psychologically. Since traumatization often occurs in the setting of fundamental (and not transient) relationships, a paradoxical situation is established in which the person responsible for traumatizing the victim is also someone charged with ensuring their psychological well-being (such as a parent, or a spouse).

As we have emphasized in the preceding discussion, fundamental relationships are crucially dependent on an ongoing capacity to offer nurturance and provide an opportunity to soothe and support the other person and keep them mobilized (parent to child, and spouses mutually). Furthermore, a good deal of that nurturance needs to be taken for granted.

There is a component of a merger in the parent/child and male/female relationship through which the other person is seen as idealizable. The parent or a spouse needs to be experienced not only in the positive light, but also as being idealizable, because, without that quality, they cannot really be a soothing presence in times of need (i.e. they cannot furnish narcissistic supplies).

Abuse (either physical or sexual or psychological) is an event, or, more commonly, a series of events which are dramatically at odds with the concept of sustained nurturance and implied connection with a benevolent figure. Such events introduce a jarring discrepancy between what is experienced and what one needs to experience to feel safe and normal. Having an abusive parent/spouse is not merely a question of dealing with a specific action, but with an underlying sense that the background of psychological safety has now been invaded or disrupted. The abused spouse /child is dislodged from a position of safety, yet they often do not have resources to leave. Thus, a chronic situation can emerge in which the victimized person is torn between two incompatible objectives: he/she continues to feel obliged to be defensive and self-protective while, at the same time, they cannot help wishing to reestablish the original merger in order to recover the basic trust and the original background of safety.

This protracted struggle (which may last for years) to both stake out a space of safety in which one is protected against the person who hurt them, while also trying to reestablish the aggressor as an idealizable figure and a source of narcissistic supplies is a work against great odds and psychologically very costly. Anger at the aggressor and blaming will naturally accompany this psychological struggle, yet these feelings can exist alongside an ongoing need to reunite psychologically with the person who hurt them.

A very active conflict is thus kept alive between the need to withdraw from the punitive parent and the need to fashion them somehow into a figure who is idealizable. A series of traumatic disappointments which are evoked in this setting can, over a long period of time, eventually lead to traumatic de-idealization.

Paradoxically, the vulnerability to traumatic de-idealization is founded in an ongoing need to have viable partners and parents. Idealizable parents are a source of narcissistic assets and supplies which support the development of the child. In a similar way, idealizable partners maintain the continuity of marriage which can be seen as a protracted developmental process in its own right and not a steady state. If a person never needed narcissistic supplies and were wholly emotionally independent, they would not be vulnerable to traumatic de-idealization.

The second factor which increases the likelihood of a traumatic de-idealization has to do with the long-term nature of fundamental relationships. They are essentially long-term and need to be long-term in order to make possible their particular developmental objectives. This in turn implies that the cumulative impact of many disappointments (instead of a single event) becomes especially relevant.

For this reason, the dynamics of traumatic de-idealization are most useful and relevant when dealing with cases of long-term post-traumatic adaptation which includes a certain number of pseudoseizure cases.

Issues of control and self-definition

In the context of traumatic de-idealization, anger (paradoxically) serves to mobilize others into an empathic stance which is meant to reestablish the bond and repair the narcissistic injury. However, anger can serve other functions in individuals who have been rendered narcissistically vulnerable.

In working with war victims, especially refugees, a paradoxical situation is sometimes encountered in which the traumatized individual not only does not welcome the relief that is offered, but may rebuff all overtures. While anger at the aggressor is, of course, completely understandable and expected in this setting, this particular anger does not seem to be explicitly concerned with or directed at the aggressor, nor is it intended to mobilize the person offering help into seeking restitution for the victim. The anger seems to have a different psychological aim, namely a function of *asserting one's identity and separateness from others.*

We may ask why this should be such an important psychological aim for the survivors. The situation of a war victim is marked by extreme narcissistic vulnerability: the victim is permeated with the traumatic sense that one is not only not an equal, one is not much at all. What has been especially injured here is the component of self-feeling which Kohut referred to as twinship—a sense that others are reassuringly like us. This is not so much an idea as it is a feeling—a way of experiencing others. This type of relatedness has a number of important implications.

The crucial component of the sense of twinship is the expectation that others are not a source of threat (since we are like them). This, in turn, implies that, if we are harmed, they will understand and respond right away, because that is how one treats those are who are equals and equal in value. Consistent with this view is a further expectation that persons in one's environment or larger community will not view the trauma as something which is just "a part of life", but will recognize it fully as a clear break in the normal course of events.

The "why me?" feelings are a very significant aspect of the situation. Although frequently brushed aside as unproductive, they are in no way a sign of immaturity, and they are not unproductive but necessary.

The "why me?" is not an absurd question. On the contrary, it is a very natural question which attests to the presence of a narcissistic bond which rests on the merger with society and which, in turn, permits the individual a baseline of feeling of safety and optimism which does not have to be reestablished and renegotiated every day. "Why me" feelings are thus neither immature nor unexpected. They reflect the nature of the bond to society, and this emotional sense implies that all individuals are equally protected. The merger not only does not permit the psychological experience of randomness in the world, its key function is to shield the individual from it. This is why the "why me?" question is often asked by traumatized individuals whether they articulate it or not.

A person who has been severely or acutely traumatized may feel different things at different stages of recovery. Being angry, especially being angry at others in the environment who are manifestly not connected with the aggressor (or may even try to help), may be a response to a profound sense that one has been stripped of the feeling of control and self-determination and that the only way to reverse this catastrophic loss is through anger.

Anger functions protectively by enforcing psychological separateness from others. It creates a wall or a shield which protects one from further narcissistic injury: If am not as good as you, *at least I am not the same* as you. Anger offers relief from a sense of traumatic anonymity.

Pseudoseizure patients

This mechanism of asserting one's identity and control through anger is not limited to war victims. It occurs in other traumatized individuals as well, including the pseudoseizure patients.

In working with pseudoseizure patients, one periodically encounters a psychological situation which is characterized by an impasse. The patient appears very contrary, may argue, engages in blaming, appears stubbornly angry, rejects empathic overtures, indeed, appears to reject any efforts to reach him (or her). He or she cannot be talked out of this angry stance. The therapist is left with the feeling that everything he or she does is wrong.

While an angry stance can occur for any number of reasons, it is helpful to consider that, for someone who was traumatized, it may serve to establish interpersonal distance, the purpose of which is to prevent further narcissistic injury.

A victim in the traumatic de-idealization situation seeks merger to repair injured self-esteem. In the latter situation, however, the victim seeks distance to prevent injury or reduce its impact. These two different functions of anger are not mutually exclusive and may occur in the same individuals at different stages of recovery.

Seeking distance through anger is not a permanent posture of traumatized individuals. It may occur in acute stages when a sense of threat is still very poignant and the individual has not had the chance to begin working on a solution. The goal of their anger is not really aggressive; its major function is to make people stop and pay attention to the fact that the person was hurt. This is not a manipulative or histrionic bid for attention. It is an attempt to prevent feelings of panic which can arise from realizing that others will simply breeze by while one is hurting.

Points of technique

The therapist can help the patient with a statement which acknowledges the patient's feeling that, right at this moment, they really do not have another way of making others pay attention to what has happened to them.

It seems that you are feeling so badly, that the only way you see of hanging on is to make someone else stop whatever they are doing and experience what you are feeling.

OR

You do not want people to simply go about their business when you feel like you are drowning. It does not seem fair that they should simply go on about their business when you are feeling this badly.

The patient may respond to this intervention in which case he or she will become more engaged, more verbal and the impasse will be lessened.

Some patients, however, may be too immobilized and find it difficult to respond verbally, or they may simply not be ready to acknowledge this motivation. In order to help them one may offer the following comment:

Right now, without knowing why and through no fault of your own, you are experiencing something which is driving you to make people stop and pay attention to what you are feeling. In the future, whenever you start feeling this way again I want you to stop and let me know so that we may look at it together. We do not need to understand it right away, but if we keep working, eventually we will.

Inducing symmetric affect as a defense

The traumatized person's need for others to stop and acknowledge—even briefly and symbolically—their traumatic experience is not an unusual response in special circumstances. Not infrequently, trauma causes a sudden realization that one is less than other people. This is an acutely painful feeling. One way of reversing this feeling promptly is to induce in the other person—even for a moment- the same feeling one is just experiencing (symmetric affect). The purpose of this psychological strategy is to reestablish narcissistic balance.

The need to elicit in others one's own traumatic affect can occur in other clinical settings, for example, in the setting of borderline regressions. In that context (as will be recalled from our earlier discussion) the need to induce traumatic affect in another person is motivated by the need to be affectively contained by them, and thereby to detoxify one's own intolerable affect. The borderline individual is unable to perform this function for himself or herself, because of a structural deficit in the capacity for self-soothing. Their way of relating is driven by the need to induce the other person to compensate for someone else's developmental deficit. The other person is thus placed in a position of providing a homeostatic function for a weak system. They are experienced as a symbolic parent with whom one seeks to merge.

This is very different from the need to induce symmetric affect as an attempt to redress narcissistic imbalance, i.e. to restore the feeling that one is no worse than anyone else.

The need to redress a narcissistic imbalance in this particular way is not a ubiquitous part of the post-traumatic response. However, it occurs with sufficient frequency to merit attention.

This dynamic pattern can be easily overlooked, because the traumatized individual may not be aware of their urge to seek relief in this particular way. What is even more likely is that they are not prepared to admit it, either to themselves or to others, and may in fact be embarrassed or ashamed of this motivation.

The need to elicit defensively the same affect in others may be satisfied simply by a brief response from the other person. It may not require a prolonged or elaborate empathic response and commitment. However, if this does not occur, elaborate regressions can sometimes be triggered in which the traumatized person becomes progressively more insistent about getting attention on a wide range of issues, or may become hostile, with displaced anger which does not, at first, make sense.

Not all clinical situations which have this chaotic and deteriorating quality are due to the activation of this need to elicit in others symmetric affect. However, this pattern occurs with sufficient frequency to merit our attention.

Bearing in mind that the patient is not able to articulate the nature of this process, nor what he or she is actually seeking, it is helpful to give the patient an opportunity to address this issue.

Narcissistic vulnerability and war victims

The significance of the social contract

The relationship between the individual and society can be viewed as one of the fundamental relationships. The concept of the social contract refers to the assumed contract between the individual and society which regulates their relationship, much as other relationships are regulated, namely by stating rights and obligations of both. The society provides nurturance and sustains the individual, creating stability and an expectation of well-being. An important part of what society provides for the individual is a protection from harm and aggression. The individual, in turn, behaves in a responsible manner with respect to the rights of others and yields some of his or her autonomy to social institutions.

The concept of social contract was formulated by Jean Jacques Rousseau (1712–1778), an 18th-century French philosopher and author. The following quotations (Rousseau, 1913) present an effort to capture some of the ideas with which Rousseau attempted to characterize the nature of the dialectic relationship between the individual and society.

> As the force and liberty of each man are the chief instruments of his self-preservation, how can he pledge them without harming his own interests, and neglecting the care he owes to himself? This difficulty, in its bearing on my present subject, may be stated in the following terms:
>
> The problem is to find a form of association which will defend and protect with the whole common force the person and goods of each associate, and in which each, while uniting himself with all, may still obey himself alone, and remain as free as before [pp. 13–14].
>
> Each of us puts his person and all his power in common under the supreme direction of the general will, and in our corporate capacity, we receive each member as an indivisible part of the whole.

> At once, in place of the individual personality of each contracting party, this act of association creates a moral and collective body, composed of as many members as the assembly contains voters, and receiving from this act its unity, its common identity, its life and its will [p. 15].

> As soon as this multitude is so united in one body, it is impossible to offend against one of the members without attacking the body, and still more to offend against the body without the members resenting it. Duty and interest therefore equally oblige the two contracting parties to give each other help [p. 17].

> What man loses by the social contract is his natural liberty and an unlimited right to everything he tries to get and succeeds in getting: what he gains is civil liberty and the proprietorship of all he possesses [p. 19].

Given this understanding of the relationship between the individual and the society, what consequences would a traumatic event have? A traumatic event disrupts the expectation of safety which the individual needs to function. Trauma represents the breaking of the contract which has occurred without the fault of the individual. There is a random or capricious quality to the breaking of the social contract which is emotionally particularly disruptive. Understandably, a good deal of resentment is frequently generated in this situation which persists if this disruption is not somehow reversed or repaired, even symbolically.

The idea of the social contract —whether explicit or implicit —is a useful framework in which to place our discussion of the reciprocal rights and obligations between an individual and society. The notion of a contract has the connotation of a rational, negotiated and conscious agreement between consenting parties. Certainly, there are areas of functioning in which the life of an individual is and needs to be organized on that level. However, to fully appreciate the nature and also the extent of psychological disturbance which can occur when this contract is broken, we need to expand our notion of the social contract to include the elements of a narcissistic bond.

I contend that the relationship between the individual and society can be viewed as one of the fundamental relationships, along with the marital partnership and the parent–child bond. This has several important implications. To begin with, it means that it shares the character of the narcissistic bond.

A narcissistic bond is crucially different in several important aspects from a usual contract. A narcissistic bond exists between partners who are *not* equals psychologically, and it can be argued that this is true, in important ways, of the relationship between the individual and society as well. I contend that the relationship between society and the individual contains a significant component of a merger (idealization, as well as twinship elements). In this merger the individual relates to society as a whole as to an idealizable parent, and to its individual members as brothers and equals.

A merger involves an implicit expectation for ongoing support and response. This element of *assumed* connection often exists alongside explicit awareness of one's obligations to society. The individual may function in his daily life as a mature, hardworking adult and a model citizen. The two levels of relatedness, however different, are not mutually exclusive—they are complementary.

The merger does not exist, because the individual is immature—it exists, because it provides the background of emotional protection in a world which is inevitably unpredictable. While societies vary dramatically in the extent to which they provide stable and safe environments, nevertheless, traumatic events eventually occur which tend to disrupt any individual person's perception of being in control which is crucial to being an equal in any situation. Thus, the nature of social life is such that any adult can be abruptly faced with events which cause him or her to regress emotionally into the position reminiscent of a child who needs to rely on a benevolent parent.

This regression need not be pervasive and it need not be permanent. Furthermore, the regression does not preclude courage and a capacity on the part of the individual to take an instrumental and problem-solving orientation towards events in one's life. Still, there is an ongoing potential for disruption present in any society which precludes anyone from being permanently secure and permanently an equal.

The presence of merger (and other elements of narcissistic relatedness), brings both advantages and disadvantages, as it does in other relationships. On the one hand, these connections provide an ongoing, rather than transient reassurance—in a sense, a psychological bridge. On the other hand, a disruption of the merger can lead to rapid regression in the person's functioning.

The breaking of the bond between the individual and society is exemplified in the most powerful way in the situation of war victims. Being subjected to a threat or a sight of mortal danger, having one's house burned and being dispossessed and set afoot is as drastic a tear in the fabric of connections which assure the life of society as one can imagine.

Wars represent an extremely explicit shattering of the assumption that one is embedded in the benevolent relationship with society. They disrupt mergers in violent ways. They force the awareness of "the other" as profoundly and dangerously different—"resembling nothing that is ours" (Poe, 2002 b).

The emotional sense that others are profoundly different is traumatic. It is not, nor is it intended to be, a part of our daily experience, rather, it is a part of traumatic experience. The feeling that others are profoundly different is really an experience of dangerous discontinuity. This discontinuity could be compared to the experience of someone who becomes suddenly aware of a crack or a fault in the cement floor on which one is standing. The crack in the cement floor is not a neutral event. It is not an event which occurs in isolation, but a rare event which signals an earthquake or other imminent disaster.

The awareness of others as profoundly different thus leads to a sense of discontinuity in our self-feeling and our experience of the world. A sense of emotional discontinuity is very close to a sense of disorganization. Thus, a discontinuity is more than just a painful feeling—it is a threat to the foundation of the self. It signals, much as the fault in the cement floor, a danger of fragmentation. Such experience readily sets off processes of narcissistic injury and narcissistic rage, as well as immobilization.

We should qualify this discussion by a comment that not all experience of war victims follows the above paradigm. It is one of the possible mechanisms of traumatogenesis. Nor do all survivors respond with the same intensity—indeed, as with other traumatic events, some individuals become defensively constricted and hardly respond at all. Still, the notion that the relationship between the individual and society is not only not casual, but of necessity bears important similarities to the so-called fundamental relationships (such at the parent/child) is useful when we try to approach the many faces of post-traumatic symptomatology. Some of the symptoms suggest strongly the character of narcissistic injury and traumatic de-idealization (as a chronic outcome). If we accept that a certain number of individuals who have been traumatized through war, assault, etc, follow the traumatic de-idealization paradigm, there is an important implication.

This has to do with the tendency of the patients, including pseudoseizure patients, to continue to struggle to reestablish the original position of safety through merger, and to continue to seek to evoke in others response and resonance that would reassure them that others are essentially like them. There is a strong urge to repair the rift and the discontinuity that trauma has engendered.

Applicability to pseudoseizure patients

Disturbances of initiative or the victim's privilege not to take action

Disturbances in initiative are common in patients with traumatically based pseudoseizures. They can be triggered by different psychological mechanism, however. They can occur as a result of the process of grieving (recalling our earlier discussion). They can also reflect an identification with the traumatized parent. In addition, they could represent a response to the breaking of the social contract. In this section, we shall explore this particular dynamic in more detail.

Disturbances of initiative are often seen in chronic cases, although they are by no means limited to them. They vary with respect to their severity and complexity. They could be mild, or very pervasive in which case they can cause a good deal of immobilization and impoverishment.

Disturbances of initiative are, in some respects, more challenging to deal with than overt symptoms. Overt symptoms such as, for example, intrusive memories, or other signs of acute distress, are explicit. They stand out clearly against the background of the patient's normal life or their usual demeanor. Problems with initiative, however, do not stand out against the background of the patient's life (unless someone is also very depressed). They are somehow embedded or integrated within the framework of the patient's life.

A certain proportion of patients with traumatically based pseudoseizures exhibit a marked constriction in their life-style. This is one of the principal manifestations of disturbed initiative in this group. One encounters a very cautious stance and a desire not to venture beyond the confines of present life parameters, even if they are far from satisfactory. It appears that some individuals reach a particular point after trauma when they have stabilized to some extent, and have evolved a life structure or routine which may be very constricted, yet which mostly works from day to day.

Here, one could properly remark that many nontraumatized individuals tend to live such lives as well, and that many people prefer not to go beyond that which has proven safe and simple for them. If such an approach to life is adopted by choice, by a more or less conscious decision, there is of course nothing wrong with it. If, however, the personality constriction is so marked that it limits the person in an unnatural or crippling way, or is occurring largely as a consequence of adaptation to trauma, then it becomes clinically significant. Pseudoseizure patients who have been traumatized rarely choose a constricted life-style. It is much more likely that they have constricted their lives defensively.

In a successful working through of traumatic experience the individual is expected to return to life again, and accept new possibilities, for better or worse, being able to tolerate some degree of risk. The opposite happens in some forms of adaptation to trauma in which there is a marked pull away from an involvement with and investment into the world. There is a strong need to maintain sameness. The patients may remain very focused on caring for their immediate or extended family, but nevertheless lead their lives in such a way that all else is more or less jettisoned. There is a reluctance to trust and to invest into personal growth. The patient may seem superficially open yet lead her life as if she were a member of a threatened species.

Why is this a problem, and for whom is it a problem? It is a problem if the motivation to maintain one's life within such a rigid framework is not based on the lack of resources or ability, but is occurring as a consequence of resentment (also fear) and other negative affects which are associated with the breaking of the social contract.

As we proposed earlier, trauma represents a breaking or a disruption of the social contract that exists between the individual and society and that binds one to the other. That contract cannot be disrupted with impunity, because it regulates how society and the individual relate to one another—not in a single situation, but permanently (i.e. their mutual regulation is normative, and not periodic).

The social contract implies mutual involvement. Mutual involvement, in turn, implies a mutual investment of energies, resources and commitment. Society invests in the individual and the individual invests in society. While the degree of mutual involvement varies markedly, the relationship between the individual and society cannot be maintained without active effort—it is not automatic. It is a homeostatic system and like all homeostatic systems, it runs on energy. The fact that it is not automatic and that it rests on the foundation of mutual investment becomes especially evident when some traumatic event takes place which creates an imbalance.

Some individuals who have been traumatized are reluctant to become involved with society again, because this feels like investing when one has been robbed. It does not make sense. In some respects, trauma feels like being mugged. No one deserves to be mugged and the person expects some form of a response or redress by society when it happens.

It is true that not everyone who has been traumatized responds in this particular way. Nevertheless, a substantial proportion of traumatized individuals feel resentment, sometimes a good deal of it, in consequence of a particular traumatic experience which befell them. Their response may be very much that of a person who was mugged. We have already explored the analogy to mugging in describing the nature of anger in individuals who have been victims of motor vehicle accidents. This analogy is equally applicable in this setting.

Victims of mugging are clearly seen as victims and there is rarely any controversy over it. Even if the perpetrator is never caught, or any money recovered, still, no one has any serious doubts as to the nature of that event. It is not, for example, characterized as "civil unrest" and no one alleges that the elderly woman was parted from her money in a consensual way. Furthermore, a mugging is not seen as an accident, or as something for which the victim is partly or totally responsible. The victim of mugging is not told that "these things happen" or that "one should get past it and get on with one's life". Trauma, on the other hand, (unless it is death of a loved one) is not necessarily seen as a loss, nor is the traumatized individual automatically perceived as someone who was de facto robbed of something.

The sense of being robbed is not based on delusional thinking, nor is it due to a sense of narcissistic entitlement although both of those reactions can also occur in some individuals who have been traumatized. There is more to this motivation than an effort to obtain disability. The sense of being robbed and the need to obtain redress stem from a more basic psychological need to repair the rupture in the implicit contract with society that was disrupted through trauma. That repair need not involve costly compensations.

Sometimes, it does not involve any material compensation at all, but rather a response from society—some kind of a gesture, or a statement which reflects the acknowledgment of the feeling that something took place which was clearly wrong.

Until this process of repair gets under way, the individual feels that he or she cannot fully trust again and does not feel right about being involved again.

We should add at this point that the sense of resentment is not a petty resentment of someone who is tightly monitoring all that is given and all that is received in some type of elaborate, ongoing book of emotional accountancy. Rather, one feels robbed of the background of safety which trauma has disrupted. If it happened suddenly once, why not again? Thus, the quality of randomness is introduced into one's life which the patient may feel helpless against and which he or she cannot dispel in any simple way. This kind of psychological situation fuels resentment.

Traumatized individuals who feel a sense of resentment and reluctance to reinvest in society may hesitate to admit such feelings to others (perhaps even to themselves) since our society very clearly does not endorse such sentiments and considers them blameworthy. Active coping with trauma, building life again—i.e. actions through which the individual *re-invests into society*—are seen as worthy and desirable. While no one questions that they are, it is equally true that a person who feels a keen sense that something was lost in a wrong way is also correct. He (or she) cannot simply wish his resentment away just because such sentiments are not admirable.

How can the clinician be helpful? The clinician can help by keeping in mind that the dynamics of broken contact with society might operate in the patient's resentment and constricted life-style.

We noted earlier that constriction might also be due to mourning or an identification with a traumatized parent. All three possibilities should be considered. There is no a priori reason why one possibility should be explored preferentially, because this depends largely on the patient's total clinical presentation and the quality of affect which is evident in the session. Complicated mourning might be considered if the clinical picture contains depressive coloring and other evidence of grief. On the other hand, if resentment and irritability are in evidence, and there is a stubborn adherence to a restricted lifestyle, this might favor the broken contract hypothesis. If the particular hypothesis, which was first pursued, proves wrong, no harm will come to the patient. It is more important that the clinician be aware that different dynamic mechanisms might operate in this picture.

Points of technique

To open up the discussion to the possibility that the patient is troubled significantly by feelings of helpless resentment is already an important step. It is not difficult to do so and, again should this line of inquiry prove incorrect, no harm will ensue. The clinician should thus have a low threshold for beginning an inquiry into the issue of the broken contract.

One can introduce the topic by a statement which acknowledges that the particular traumatic event which occurred was not all right, and that it would be natural to feel very frustrated. The purpose of this statement is not to tell the patient what they are feeling, but to suggest that it would be natural to feel upset or resentful in such a situation. In other words, to acknowledge that such affects would be appropriate in such a context, and that the therapist would not be disappointed or think less of the patient for having them. In particular, the statement is meant to communicate that the therapist does not consider the patient immature or blameworthy for experiencing affects which society does not endorse. This intervention creates an opening, a space for dialogue for this important issue.

The therapist may explore the issue further by stating how disruptive a particular event or circumstance must have been and asking the patient how they are going about putting their life back together, acknowledging for example, that it might take a lot of work. This is a supportive statement which acknowledges that the therapist understands that it takes work to recover, and that it does not simply happen automatically. In other words, recovery costs something. The notion of cost creates a therapeutic bridge to the feelings of resentment.

Narcissistic injury and postconcussive syndrome

Minor head trauma often has numerous adverse consequences which amount to a series of losses in the injured person's emotional, cognitive, and social functioning (as discussed in Section I of this book). A certain (not insubstantial) proportion of these patients have an unfavorable outcome with ongoing impairment leading to a loss of occupational role. An ongoing impairment of sufficient magnitude to cause a loss of competitive employment is probably the most damaging aspect of the situation, as it amounts to a traumatic disruption of both one's social role and one's social identity.

The clinical picture of head trauma and its consequences, especially its chronic sequelae, is very complex. From the standpoint of a clinician (psychologist, neurologist, psychiatrist) trying to understand psychological reactions to trauma, and, especially, chronic adaptation to trauma and its psychological cost to the patient, the concepts of narcissistic loss and narcissistic injury are especially relevant.

Narcissistic losses/injuries refer to situations in which a person has been rendered significantly narcissistically vulnerable. This experience of vulnerability often has an acute onset, and is marked by an abrupt loss of the sense of vitality, pride, security or personal initiative and effectiveness, leading to a sense of acute resentment, anger and shame which may or may not be expressed.

Narcissistic losses are not just drops in self-esteem; they are characterized by a peculiar sense of being abruptly deprived of something which is rightfully one's own, something which can be counted on and which, in fact, forms a background of normal experience and is, therefore, unalienable. In a narcissistic loss/injury there is a sudden traumatic realization of a disruption in this background of normal experience and self-feeling. There is an element of being rudely surprised such as might occur in a person who (literally) had a rug pulled from under them, or a person who finds that all his clothes have unaccountably disappeared, or a person who stumbles.

Patients who have suffered a minor/moderate head trauma and have developed a postconcussive/post-traumatic syndrome have narcissistic injury at several levels and in several life domains. One of these important domains is the area of neuropsychological functioning.

A number of patients have persistent neuropsychological disturbances such as unreliable attention, concentration and memory. The cumulative effect of these and similar cognitive deficits is a diminished sense of cognitive control which is a great deal more disruptive than being troubled by a single well-defined problem. Becoming aware of these deficits can be acutely painful and disorganizing even when the deficits are characterized as mild by a formal evaluation.

Kohut (1972, p. 383) described the nature of narcissistic loss and rage in the following terms:

> His rage is due to the fact that he is suddenly not in control of his own thought processes, a function which people consider to be most intimately their own – i.e., as a part of the self. "It must not be! It cannot be! Our thought processes are taken by us as belonging to the core of our self, and we refuse to admit that we may not be in control of them. To be deprived of the capacity to name a familiar object or to solve a simple problem is experienced as more incredible than even the loss of a limb. Our own body can be seen and, since perception is primarily directed toward the outside world, it is easier to think of our body in objective terms. The unseeable thought processes, however, are considered by us as inseparable from, or coinciding with, our very self. The loss of a limb can therefore be mourned, like the loss of a love object; a defect in the realm of our mental functions, however, is experienced as a loss of self.

We should add in this context that Kohut did not deal with pseudoseizure patients and the above description does not refer to them. However, the above depiction of the nature of narcissistic injury conveys the meaning of the experience in a remarkable way and is very applicable to pseudoseizure cases with a history of head trauma.

The experience of narcissistic loss involves a sense of primitive preverbal panic; it is not a well-formulated response to a well-defined problem. From the standpoint of the patient, neuropsychological deficits are neither clear nor well-defined.

From the point of view of a clinician (or a family member), the patient's inability to remember a name, or recall the order of a series of appointments may seem like a clear-cut deficit, but it really is not. Memory, attention, mental flexibility, etc. are clinical terms which help the clinician in organizing his thinking about the patient's problems, and as such are necessary. However, these processes are not really well understood and, from the point of view of the patient's subjective experience, they cover a great deal of ground.

The patient who cannot remember a name, or cannot do something which was perfectly simple until very recently is not really dealing psychologically with a specific deficit. His emotional response is not to a specific deficit, but, rather, to the fact that there has been a weird *intrusion into* the world of *his customary experience,* and that (if only for a brief moment) things are definitely not normal.

It could be argued that not being able to retrieve a word at a particular moment (to use but a simplest example) is not, by itself, a matter of dire consequence. No permanent harm is likely to occur if it is remembered half a day later. However, it is not that a particular word is important as such, but being able to perform this task automatically and not with special effort and a delay.

"Blips" of abnormal experience need not deal with dramatic phenomena (such as command hallucinations) to be disturbing. They need not be long and the person may eventually recover. However, the fact that they occur at all makes them disturbing, especially if they occur several times a day, and are both unpredictable and chronic which is a pattern frequently described by patients with postconcussive/posttraumatic syndrome. They create a situation which could be conceptualized as "a disturbed baseline", "a deteriorating baseline", or a "drifting baseline".

In a "drifting" baseline, small failures to perform at the customary levels are interspersed throughout the day so that a task may be performed automatically and effortlessly on one occasion, but not on another. The patient has no means of knowing whether he will recover his previous baseline (i.e., his normal experience and functioning), and he does not really know what is happening to him.

In the setting of a neuropsychological evaluation, a patient may perform in an impaired range on a specific memory or concentration item which is interpreted as a specific deficit and seems relatively straightforward. Again, from the standpoint of the patient's experience, the deficit is not nearly as circumscribed and it is certainly not straightforward. Having a name for a deficit helps, however, that is only the first step. A name, even a useful description, does not provide the patient with all he needs to take on the problem, nor does it tell him when the disturbance will begin or end.

If his baseline of cognitive functioning is sufficiently disrupted, it is this disruption per se which may trigger a sense of traumatic loss. This sense of traumatic loss, in turn, does not reflect a loss of a specific function (like concentration), but a threat to the loss of self. To experience such a threat can be very disorganizing. The patient may respond to the threat by a brief panic reaction in which despair, shame and rage are mixed. During this reaction which may seem out of proportion to the nature of the deficit, the patient may not be easy to reach and console. Also, the patient cannot be argued out of this state. However, appreciating the nature of the narcissistic loss can help the clinician be patient and empathic toward the patient who needs to be allowed time to recover and resume the evaluation in a manner which is comfortable to him or her.

Understanding the role of narcissistic loss in cognitive deficits following head injury is important, because this loss can strike hard at the sense of self and damage self-cohesion. This is not the same as merely stating that emotional problems are common after head injury, or that the patient has problems with impulse control. Although that is certainly often true, a great deal more is involved than being volatile or impulsive. Unpredictable, yet persisting problems with memory, concentration or mental flexibility create a *background of disturbance and deviation* from the patient's average expectable environment.

We might argue that a state in which a cognitive deficit is manifest (for example, a patient cannot retrieve a word) is experientially a different state from the one in which he feels in control and functions as usual (or at pre-morbid levels). Instances of cognitive deficit are thus instances of intrusions of different states into the experiential baseline. These instances may be brief, but having to recover from them is very disruptive and tiring. They create of background of frequent "state transitions" (to borrow the term from EEG) which may resemble restless sleep disrupted by brief episodes of wakefulness. We may compare the patient whose experiential baseline is daily disrupted by episodes of cognitive deficit to a patient with a sleep disturbance whose sleep is fragmented by episodes of arousal. These episodes may or may not lead to wakefulness, but they disrupt the sleep significantly and they reduce its restorative character. Clinicians who deal with insomnia (as well as other forms of sleep pathology) use an index of disruption which includes total amount of wakefulness after sleep onset (WASO) (Carscadon and Rechtschaffen, in Kryger, Roth and Dement, 2000, p. 1197).

Using the analogy to sleep disturbance, we might argue that a similar index could be developed to reflect the extent of disruption caused by the intrusion of episodes of cognitive deficit into the background of normal awareness. The disruptive nature of neuropsychological deficits is reflected not only in the total number of episodes, but also in the fact that these episodes represent transitions in the experiential state. State transitions, in turn, require adaptation—recovery does not occur automatically. An index of disruption would help underscore the extent to which even the so-called mild cognitive deficits disrupt the daily life of a patient. It is one thing to say that the patient has ongoing deficits, it is quite another to say that during his waking hours he has experienced 8 state transitions, each requiring some effort to recover.

Earlier in our discussion, we noted that patients with a post-concussive/post-traumatic syndrome associated with pseudoseizures experience narcissistic losses in several domains of life or at several levels of functioning. In addition to the narcissistic injury related to cognitive deficits, there is the more comprehensive level of loss related to the loss of employment with the associated financial uncertainty, a sense of not bringing closure to one's life, and many other issues (as discussed in Section I of this book).

These are not issues which tend to disappear. They require ongoing attention and struggle (the chronic level of narcissistic loss). In the acute form, narcissistic injury is an intensely painful, driven state and the patient feels an intense pressure to be out of it. A sense of shame is a particularly painful aspect of narcissistic injury and a special challenge to deal with. Anger or externalization of blame are common narcissistic defenses against that experience.

A repeated cycle of feeling injured and being angry, helpless and ashamed, as a response to it, is psychologically costly, and very difficult to endure in the long run. Thus, a long-term adaptation occurs which can take several routes. One of them is a process of defense in which much of this material relating to the acute experiences of narcissistic injury and the associated anger/shame is submerged and repressed. I conceptualize pseudoseizures in this context as part of this defense strategy to contain intolerable affects related mainly to narcissistic loss (often chronic levels of narcissistic loss) and conflicts which exist at several levels.

Special topics in the diagnosis and management of pseudoseizures

The initial presentation of the findings of a pseudoseizure evaluation to the patient is a clinical situation which may seem very routine and straightforward. While it is certainly routine, it is not straightforward from the psychological point of view.

It can mobilize several difficult issues which may adversely affect the future management of the case. These issues have to do with the meaning of pseudoseizures to both the physician and the patient, as well as with the physician's readiness to deal with certain types of material which the patient brings and which cannot be classified as symptoms. Yet another important issue which can arise in this setting has to do with an expectation that patients with pseudoseizures—not having a lesional disorder of the central nervous system—will be able to improve on their own as a matter of course.

The dynamic issues discussed in this section are chiefly relevant to the neurologist. The sensitivity to these issues can facilitate greatly the success of the initial presentation of diagnostic findings to the patient, as well as assist in establishing a therapeutic alliance which is crucial for follow-up.

The topics which are explored in the following sections are concerned, to a large extent, with issues of narcissistic vulnerability. It is, of course, not intuitively obvious why or how a particular attitude toward pseudoseizures might trigger narcissistic vulnerability in the patient. In the following sections we shall make an attempt to demonstrate how this particular dynamics operates. Sensitivity to this issue can go a long way in averting negative patient reactions which can occur in this setting.

Narcissistic vulnerability and the meaning of pseudoseizures

The clinical definition of pseudoseizures seems straightforward once an adequate evaluation has been completed. From the standpoint of the patient who has been so diagnosed, however, matters are not so simple, and the diagnosis can raise as many issues as it resolves. We should qualify this observation by pointing out that patients respond differently to this diagnosis. We are concerned here specifically with a subset of patients for whom this diagnosis presents a difficulty and may even pose a narcissistic threat.

Whether or not the diagnosis of pseudoseizures poses a narcissistic threat depends on several factors. An especially important one is the manner in which the diagnosis is initially related to the patient. Typically, the initial diagnosis occurs after an extensive assessment in an in-patient setting in which a seizure disorder is ruled out (or, in cases of concurrent epilepsy, is not responsible for particular spells under study).

The fact that the patient does not have epilepsy, which is potentially a very disruptive disorder of the central nervous system (CNS), is a very favorable finding which should come as a relief to all concerned. However, if the neurologist conceptualizes a seizure disorder as a legitimate disorder and regards pseudoseizures as a pseudo-disorder or a bogus disorder, instead of being a *different* disorder, then he will not communicate a sense of relief that the patient fortunately does not have epilepsy. He will communicate that the patient has something counterfeit instead. Something which is, from the point of view of medical science, suspect.

This is, of course, in no way true. Pseudoseizure syndromes are not a pseudo-disorder. They are a genuine neuropsychiatric disorder, a great deal of which is understandable in terms of well-described (although perhaps not widely known) psychodynamic and neuropsychological mechanisms.

If this sense of "illegitimacy" is communicated to the patient (even unwittingly), it can easily set up a foundation for a great deal of difficulty with respect to the future management of the disorder, or the patient may simply never come back. It should be pointed out that the clinician need not state his doubts about the legitimacy of the disorder explicitly. However, if he does not believe pseudoseizures to be a legitimate disorder, he is liable to communicate his doubts to the patient, sometimes in subtle ways. This communication has several adverse consequences.

From the standpoint of the patient, it is but a short step psychologically from the idea that his disorder is suspect or not quite genuine to the idea that he, the patient, is somehow suspect as well and, therefore, is not a genuine patient. The patient, as a result, feels like an impostor and his task, psychologically, at this point, will be to prove that he is not an impostor, which is not what the patient just diagnosed should be doing at all.

A parallel psychological process is likely to occur in the neurologist. He or she is obliged to deal with a disorder which has physical manifestations, sometimes very dramatic, but not a physical illness (based on a lesion) to go with it. As a responsible physician, his (or her) primary task and first priority is to rule out a possible CNS disorder. Even after this has been ruled out by an extensive evaluation, there may remain a lingering doubt that something was missed, or worse, that a CNS disorder can never really be ruled out in the future either, with complete confidence. Thus, he is facing a situation which promises no real closure and which carries with it a threat of failure. Not being able to discover the underlying CNS (lesional) pathology can make the neurologist feel like an impostor also, because the ability to perform that specific task is the unique contribution of his profession to medical science and is also one of the key aspects of his professional self-definition.

A peculiar dynamic pattern is now established between the patient and the doctor. We may refer to this dynamic pattern as a "*double impostor scenario*".

The patient fears that the doctor is somehow going to expose him or her as someone who is not a bona fide patient, who is indeed a fraud. The doctor, in turn, fears that the patient's disorder will make him miss an important underlying lesion and thus expose him as a poor clinician.

This is more than a usual fear of failure, or a fear that one will not be able to help the patient, (although this may be a part of it). There is a fear of this particular failure of missing a lesion which calls into question the clinician's worth in a much more poignant way than a therapeutic failure (which is clearly understood to depend on a variety of other factors, and is by no means a reflection of his worth alone).

A situation of this kind makes the clinician vulnerable to experiencing not just fear, but shame. This affective state is far more difficult to manage psychologically (as are the defenses which it initiates), considerably more difficult than fear. Anger is a common psychological defense against the feeling of shame—whether it is expressed or not.

The patient's situation is very similar. Not being considered a genuine patient can easily lead to feelings of shame which can, in turn, trigger anger or a depressive withdrawal which are common mechanisms for handling feelings of shame.

The interpersonal situation depicted above deals with issues which are not minor disagreements about details of a procedure or scheduling issues. It deals with issues that affect the sense of worth of each individual and the sense that they are viable in their respective roles. The situation has a significant potential for eliciting shame and defensive anger. This combination of psychodynamic issues is very characteristic of narcissistic injury. We can thus conceptualize the situation as one in which both the doctor and the patient see in each other a source of narcissistic threat.

Seeing the patient as a source of narcissistic threat, in addition to being intensely uncomfortable, is also likely to interfere with a natural therapeutic attitude that the doctor would otherwise not hesitate to adopt. Instead of the usual empathic and supportive stance, the doctor may approach the patient with mistrust and caution. This can be traumatic to the patient who needs to be able to rely on the physician in order to obtain orientation and some degree of closure in dealing with a disorder which is complex and full of uncertainty for the patient as well. Thus, he or she needs the clinician's ongoing interest and enthusiasm, and does not want him to withdraw, either psychologically or literally.

The painful therapeutic impasse described in the "double impostor scenario" is quite avoidable. It can be avoided by being aware of specific issues in this clinical situation which can evoke a sense of narcissistic threat. The relevant points are summarized in the following terms:

Not having epilepsy should be presented as a favorable finding and definitely good news. (I am very pleased, (relieved, etc.), as I am sure we all are, to be able to tell you that you do not have epilepsy. This comes as a relief.)

To say "there is nothing physically wrong with you", although it may seem innocuous enough, is not a good way to present the findings in this context although it might be enormously reassuring to a patient fearing cancer. There are several reasons for this. It communicates, (or can be interpreted by the patient as communicating), perhaps in a subtle way, disapproval of the patient. It suggests that there is something not quite right with "having nothing physically wrong", and that the patient, in order to qualify as a bona fide patient, should have different findings, or even that all those expensive and extensive evaluations have been wasted because they yielded "no real findings". It can also communicate that the patient has no right to have his particular symptoms in the absence of "something physically wrong". If, on the other hand, one said cordially and with an air of obvious pleasure "I am delighted to say that there is nothing physically wrong" that would communicate relief and pleasure that the patient is all right which is an entirely different situation from the psychological point of view.

It is helpful to give the patient the idea that his/her symptoms are a part of the disorder which is by no means unusual, and which can be understood and treated. Which particular details the clinician chooses to include in his initial presentation of the diagnosis to the patient is, of course, a matter of his preferred technique. However, regardless of the specific wording employed, it is important to communicate to the patient that his or her disorder is genuine, often seen in clinical practice, understandable and treatable. One does not need to be an expert on this disorder to communicate those important points to the patient. They are a summary of issues around which the patient needs reassurance. He or she is baffled by what frequently turns out to have been a long battle with unsettling symptoms (pseudoseizure patients who are evaluated in tertiary settings often have a long latency between the diagnosis and the initial onset of symptoms).

The patient needs to know that his or her symptoms are not a confusing mélange of weird events and spells which no one has heard of until this particular case, that the symptoms belong to a meaningful clinical entity, and that there are professionals who understand and treat that disorder.

Communicating the sense that one is dealing with a legitimate and recognized disorder is a crucial element in presenting the findings in a therapeutic rather than a potentially traumatic way. This is the best protection against eliciting a sense of mutual narcissistic threat. Communicating such a point need not be long or elaborate and may require no more than several sentences.

The neurologist is not obliged to address all aspects of the pseudoseizure syndromes in the initial presentation of the findings. Answering honestly with "I do not know" to any question he or she is not comfortable addressing is entirely appropriate and keeps the clinician within the therapeutic framework. Neither is he (or she) called upon to address any controversial issues about this disorder in the initial presentation of the findings. He may however, state that "these are all important issues and if you wish, I can arrange for you to see Dr. H. who is a psychologist and will be able to address them".

Not all negative reactions to the initial diagnosis of pseudoseizures can be traced to the feeling or a belief on the part of the physician that pseudoseizures are not a genuine disorder.

The diagnosis of pseudoseizures can elicit such reactions, in and of itself, if it poses a narcissistic threat to the patient. Some male patients, for example, (although this is not limited to them) may experience the diagnosis of pseudoseizures as a proof of their weakness. The idea that emotional factors play a role in this particular disorder may be especially threatening and unacceptable. They also find it difficult to accept all their symptoms and difficulties in the absence of a clear physical disorder. They may be struggling to determine if their disorder is *genuine or not*.

The above issues have a strong potential for eliciting a sense of shame. Abrupt negative reactions are thus highly likely to be related to the feelings of shame.

If the patient has responded negatively to the diagnosis of pseudoseizures, an attempt should be made to help him. Referral to a psychologist would be indicated in this situation with the goal of helping explore why the patient has responded in this particular way. This effort may take several sessions. In the course of these sessions the patient would be "debriefed" as to the nature of pseudoseizures and provided with a picture of this disorder which is not narcissistically threatening.

Getting on with one's life in the setting of post-traumatic pseudoseizures

A patient who has been newly diagnosed with pseudoseizures and whose traumatic background has been revealed in the process of diagnostic evaluation is vulnerable to feelings of embarrassment. Sometimes, in this particular context, the physician who relates the diagnosis may communicate to the patient that, now that epilepsy has been satisfactorily ruled out, the patient should simply get on with their life and not dwell on the past.

From the patient's point of view, matters are not so simple, and he or she is not likely to follow this advice as a matter of course. This resistance has valid reasons and we shall attempt to account for them in this section.

While being told that they do not have epilepsy is a very important, indeed a critical step, it does not, by itself, in any way relieve the patient of the burden of his or her traumatic background. The challenge of dealing with that background is still very much ahead of them. The patient cannot simply get on with the business of living as if trauma had not occurred. What is even more important, the patient often *does not want to simply get on with their life* as if nothing had happened to them. The dynamics of the broken contract do not permit him or her to do this.

In our earlier discussion, we presented a view that the relationship between the individual and society can be conceptualized as an implicit contract. This contract does not refer to any explicit idea on the part of an individual. Rather, it presents an overall background of feeling oneself as a part of a group – a background which includes an expectation that one belongs and will be protected from harm. In exchange for the feelings of safety, the individual offers loyalty to the group.

Trauma could be conceptualized as a breaking of the implicit contract which links the individual to society. This traumatic break is accompanied by affects of resentment and helplessness.

Getting on with one's life runs counter to the affects of the broken contract. From the patient's point of view, it essentially amounts to continuing to give and invest when, in actuality, one feels deprived. The underlying feeling has to do with the need for the society to make good on the damage and adversity which trauma brought to the patient *and not the patient having to perform this task for himself.*

In this situation, we are dealing much more with the patient's motivation and affective grounding than with his or her conscious points of view. The patient is not simply getting on with his life, not because his world view prevents him, but because *it does not feel right*.

We should point out that the statements such as "you should put the past behind you and get on with your life" are not intrinsically wrong. They are well-intentioned and there are many clinical situations in which they are taken at face value as straightforward expressions of good will and support. In fact, there are circumstances such as, for example, after serious or life threatening injuries, strokes etc where such statements can communicate the physician's faith in the patient and his recovery. Such statements can thus mobilize the patient and achieve remarkable results.

However, traumatized individuals are a group of patients with special dynamics and special sensitivities. For this reason, a pseudoseizure patient may hear such statements very differently, as if one had said: You should be able to get on with your life and there is something fundamentally wrong with you if you do not.

It should be pointed out that the clinician who is relating the diagnosis of pseudoseizures to the patient (usually a neurologist) is not obliged to deal with the traumatic background of the patient's life directly or by himself. This problem is usually dealt with by a referral for psychotherapy to a psychologist or a psychiatrist or an experienced social worker. However, to *acknowledge* that the patient has had a traumatic life *is an intervention* in its own right, as it conveys an appreciation and not a denial of the impact of the patient's particular historic background.

Statements which somehow communicate that the patient should be able to get their traumatic life behind them—as a matter of course—are also interventions, although they are mostly not recognized as such. These interventions could be experienced by the patient as trivializing—albeit unintentionally—the impact on the patient of the particular traumatic events which they suffered through.

It should be pointed out that the resistance to just getting on with one's life—as a matter of course—is an indirect manifestation of the broken contract. The patient is not likely to state this resistance explicitly and, even if they appear angry, they may attribute the anger to some other cause (via displacement) perhaps to some specific hardship in their life, but not to the central issue.

The likelihood of the above manifestations of the broken contract and similar difficulties will be greatly attenuated if the clinician maintains an attitude of clear appreciation for the traumatic background of the patient's life and all the efforts he or she was obliged to undertake in order to counteract the impact of the trauma. Appreciation for the difficulty and for the patient's attempts to find his or her way among them is a symbolic repair of the broken contract.

The difference between symptom and experience

This is not merely a semantic distinction—rather it is a conceptual distinction which has practical significance, both in the initial diagnostic work-up, as well as in the long-term follow-up and treatment of pseudoseizures.

Patient complaints which come to the attention of a neurologist are highly variable in terms of their nature and etiology. Regardless of their nature, however, complaints tend to be perceived as symptoms or, at least, as potential symptoms. Neurologists share with other physicians the serious pragmatic task of determining the significance of various aspects of the material which the patient brings in and establishing which of those complaints are symptoms and which are not.

However, a certain proportion of complaints which the neurologist is likely to encounter cannot be classified as symptoms. In this situation, the physician is faced with material which has an indeterminate status. This indeterminate status is uncomfortable as it raises the anxiety that a genuine disorder/illness has been overlooked.

When evaluating the material which the patient provides it is helpful to consider the distinction between a symptom and an experience. An experience is a neutral term which permits the physician to accommodate a great variety of different subjective phenomena. This ensures a very flexible stance.

Physicians are of course trained to recognize symptoms, and it is thus natural that they should expect to find in the patient's complaints the material which can be translated into symptoms. Obtaining the patient's history has a very definite pragmatic aim, namely to elicit symptoms which will lead to a specific diagnosis which, in turn, will lead to a concrete therapeutic intervention. If the material which is elicited is not readily classifiable, a disturbing uncertainty is introduced into the diagnostic process. This fear is based on an assumption that the clinical material which cannot be properly classified probably cannot be brought under control.

Should the patient continue to report experiences which cannot be converted into symptoms, an anxiety-provoking situation can become established where the physician eventually fears hearing about experiences which cannot be easily classified. This fear is unnecessary.

There are several points to consider which are helpful in reducing the uncertainty produced by this situation.

Eliciting the material which cannot be converted into symptoms is not an exception in neurologic practice. On the contrary, it is very common, especially when dealing with patients who present with pseudoseizures, as well as patients with postconcussive syndromes and other sequelae of traumatic brain injury.

The emergence of such material is not due to the inadequacy of history taking, but to the fact that a great deal of material which exists in the consciousness, especially after head trauma or in the context of other neuropsychiatric syndromes, is not readily verbalizable and cannot be accounted for easily.

When faced with the material which is not a symptom there is a temptation to deny it, to call into question the genuineness of such an experience, or to attribute it to malingering, secondary gain, or otherwise "make it go away". Questioning the genuineness of the patient's experience is not an answer to any therapeutic problem. It does not make the experience go away.

It should be pointed out that the patient does not report experiences which are difficult to classify in order to baffle the physician. Some of those experiences may feel perfectly natural to the patient—a part of his daily baseline. Others might feel odd and may be as puzzling to the patient as they are to the physician. In either case, these are not experiences over which the patient is likely to have much control.

At this juncture, it is helpful to consider that the neurologist is not responsible for the totality of the material which the patient brings (and neither is, for that matter, the patient). The neurologist is responsible for doing the best job he or she can.

If, after an extensive diagnostic process, he has ruled out all he can, and there still remains a residue of the material not accounted for, he should accept that the patient has *experiences* which are not symptoms. These experiences need not be reduced to something else. They should not be treated as something which must be reformulated at all cost.

However, they should be acknowledged so that the patient is not made to feel that there is something wrong or even suspect in having them. These experiences may or may not be susceptible to change, but they should not be disputed. Not disputing someone's experience is in and of itself a valuable intervention.

It would be preferable, of course, if we understood the full meaning of such experiences. It is very natural to strive for closure in the diagnostic process as well as in treatment. Neither is the presence of experiences which cannot be readily accounted for or verbalized limited to clinical settings. For example, subjective experience of normal individuals also contains material which is by no means clear or verbalizable.

Acknowledging the experience is an appropriate first intervention. The next step is follow-up. Pseudoseizure patients are usually followed by a neurologist in order to ensure that a seizure disorder (or some other disorder of the nervous system) is not missed. This follow-up provides a natural context for keeping track of experiences which were of concern to the clinician. Follow-up is also a powerful method of reducing anxiety in a variety of conditions which are ambiguous and uncertain.

Why should we be concerned with the issue of uncertainty and attempt to manage it? Uncertainty plays a significant role in a number of clinical conditions. In addition to pseudoseizures, it also plays a role in epilepsy and pain syndromes.

When faced with uncertainty in the patient the physician can adopt several approaches. The first approach consists in providing as much clarity for the patient as possible (the interpretive emphasis). This works well in situations when one knows a good deal about a disorder or how it will behave, for example, how pneumonia will behave given antibiotics. Also, providing an interpretation of some specific dynamic issue which is very troubling to the patient and of which the patient may be totally unaware, for example: anniversary reactions following a loss and complicated mourning, or recurring depressions which do not respond to treatment because they are really driven by a very active conflict of which the patient is again unaware.

Although a good deal is known about pseudoseizures, nonetheless, the issue of their future course is much less clear and straightforward. In this situation, the uncertainty is managed by accepting it, while reducing its open-ended character through appointments at regular intervals (the containment emphasis). The physician is thus replacing a very open-ended timeline with a framework consisting of many short steps. This is a very significant positive intervention, because it changes the scope of the patient's responsibility to a much more manageable level, namely, until his or her next appointment.

We might describe this as the process of "grading uncertainty". The structure of psychotherapy sessions takes advantage of just this particular process, as it is clearly understood that psychodynamic issues require time for resolution.

The process of grading uncertainty is helpful in managing yet another aspect of pseudoseizures. Pseudoseizures share with epilepsy and certain types of pain conditions (nerve or neuralgic pain) the paroxysmal nature of episodes. The abrupt and unpredictable character of attacks, even if mild, is an added hardship here as it undermines the patient's sense of control. The knowledge that one has a series of follow-up appointments (which constitutes a plan) tends to ameliorate to some extent the feeling of loss of control as it serves to reinstate a sense of personal initiative.

Section III
The Model

Introduction

The purpose of this section is to introduce a model of post-traumatic disturbance such as is likely to occur in pseudoseizure patients. This model summarizes key elements of our earlier discussions.

Post-traumatic syndromes of pseudoseizure patients exist on a large continuum of post-traumatic syndromes of which classical post-traumatic stress disorder (PTSD) is only one variant. Pseudoseizure patients frequently present with complex, partial or chronic variants of PTSD. In the following sections we will attempt to summarize the nature of post-traumatic disturbance, as well as the nature of trauma.

Traumatic disturbance in pseudoseizure patients

- Prevalence
- Persistence (chronicity)
- Protean symptom picture

Prevalence

How prevalent are post-traumatic syndromes? This question should probably be more aptly phrased in the following way. Are post-traumatic syndromes which include partial, complex and chronic forms—and not just the classic PTSD—sufficiently common in clinical settings to be relevant? The answer to this question is "yes". They are sufficiently common to make a difference. Consequently, when evaluating and treating patients with pseudoseizures, the clinician should not hesitate to inquire about the history of trauma/loss.

Persistence (chronicity)

We do not know what percentage of pseudoseizures arise acutely, i.e. in the immediate aftermath of traumatic events. Dissociation can occur acutely in the setting of extreme events (battlefield, sexual assault) where it serves to provide immediate defense against terror and disorganization.

However, pseudoseizure episodes which are a part of a disorder or a syndrome are more than dissociation. They are an ongoing, not just a momentary defense against some traumatic experience. Their presence indicates an unresolved trauma. Pseudoseizures are both a symptom and an effort to struggle with a traumatic experience. Recurrence of pseudoseizures constitutes, in and of itself, chronicity.

The latency between trauma and the onset of pseudoseizures is very difficult to establish with precision, particularly when evaluating adult patients. "Newly diagnosed" pseudoseizures does not imply "recent-onset" pseudoseizures. When evaluating newly diagnosed patients we cannot state with certainty whether their disorder is new or not. This is especially true of patients whose trauma is related to childhood abuse. It is very possible that the traumatic disturbance is likely to be chronic, regardless of when pseudoseizures themselves began.

For patients whose pseudoseizures occur in the context of the post-traumatic/postconcussive syndrome the latency between the traumatic event (i.e. car accident) and the onset of pseudoseizures is easier to establish.

Traumatic disturbance which leads to the development of pseudoseizure syndromes is often chronic. Chronicity of traumatic disturbance, however, does not imply that pseudoseizures themselves will continue to have a chronic course. Pseudoseizures are a treatable disorder. Traumatic experiences in general, and pseudoseizures in particular, are treatable.

Untreated trauma, however, has a lengthy course in many cases. This is not surprising insofar as other disorders which remain untreated also have a difficult and lengthy course.

This is not inevitable. Early recognition and treatment of traumatic experiences is particularly important as a deterrent to the development of entrenched symptomatology which includes pseudoseizures.

Chronicity is a possible clue to trauma.

Protean symptom picture

In addition to being prevalent, post-traumatic syndromes tend to have a protean nature. This is true of PTSD in general, as well as traumatic syndromes in pseudoseizure cases.

Proteus was a minor deity from Greek mythology—a god of the sea—known for his capacity to change shape. The term "protean" has thus come to denote something which exists in many forms or manifestations and has a propensity to change.

How are post-traumatic syndromes "protean"?

They are highly comorbid with other psychiatric disorders. There is a growing consensus that PTSD is highly comorbid with other psychiatric diagnoses/conditions (Kessler et al., 1995; Breslau et al., 1997). In a sample of pseudoseizure patients of whom 88% had been victims of a traumatic experience, Bowman reported the mean of 3.1 psychiatric diagnoses per patient (Bowman, 1993).

I take the view that the co-morbid conditions are not really co-morbid, but are simply manifold manifestations of the primary traumatic disturbance. This disturbance can generate different psychiatric disorders in different patients. It can also generate different conditions/symptoms in the same patient over time. This disorder can thus not only create manifold manifestations, but these manifestations can vary from patient to patient and from time to time.

Faced with this complex picture we can ask a number of questions. One of the most obvious questions has to do with why trauma generates different psychiatric presentations. We do not have an exact answer to this question. We cannot establish with certainty why some pseudoseizure patients who have been traumatized will respond with an acute narcissistic injury and become angry and immobilized, whereas others will become withdrawn and apathetic, while still others exhibit regressions in functioning to the level of borderline syndromes. My work, however, shows that they can respond in these particular ways and it is helpful to know that.

We know that different people respond to trauma in different ways and that the final outcome, in terms of someone's overall adaptation, depends on a variety of factors, including their internal resources, their particular psychodynamic structure with both its assets and liabilities, their health and external supports, to name but a few. This position, stated in such general terms, seems like a truism which no one would dispute. It simply states the classical dictum that a particular form of adaptation or a particular response reflects some form of interaction between the individual and the environment.

The variety of manifestations of post-traumatic adaptation which we commonly encounter in clinical settings is consistent with the above dictum. We would *expect considerable differences* among individuals in response to trauma and not only one highly specific clinical course with highly specific manifestations. Yet, when dealing with post-traumatic disorders in practice this latter expectation often prevails—a belief (often unstated) that every patient will follow a clinical course of the classical PTSD, as defined by Diagnostic and Statistical Manual of Mental Disorders (DSM-IV, 1994) criteria, and exhibit a narrow range of manifestations.

Why is this belief a problem? It is a problem, because it encourages the clinician to dismiss a good deal of important information about the patient's life and to assume that the trauma had no significant impact, because it did not have this particular impact, or this particular course.

DSM-IV has excellent criteria for PTSD (American Psychiatric Association, 1994, pp. 427–9). These criteria are presented in Table 2. This description brings together symptoms which relate to traumatic re-experiencing on the one hand, and symptoms which represent numbing and withdrawal. These are seemingly totally different processes and their linkage in the diagnostic formulation reflects an important understanding based on the experience of many clinicians. It is an achievement in its own right.

The description of symptomatology is very valuable. However, it contains not only different symptoms, but different classes of symptoms. Not all symptoms are equally distinct. Flashbacks and nightmares are the hallmark symptoms of PTSD. These symptoms are dramatic and very distinct. They are high-definition symptoms by which this disorder is mostly known. They are easy to recognize. Because of their eruptive and paroxysmal nature, they attract attention. The suffering which is reflected in these symptoms is very obvious and has a strong capacity to compel therapeutic attention and intervention.

The symptoms in the second group which relate to numbing, avoidance and detachment are not nearly so distinct. Unless the patient is overtly anxious, it is not easy to determine whether they have really withdrawn and to what extent their present behavior represents detachment.

Table 2: Diagnostic criteria for 309.81 Post-traumatic Stress Disorder

A. The person has been exposed to a traumatic event in which both of the following were present:

   1. The person experienced, witnessed, or was confronted with an event or events that involved actual or threatened death or serious injury, or a threat to the physical integrity of self or others.
   2. The person's response involved intense fear, helplessness, or horror. **Note:** In children, this may be expressed instead by disorganized or agitated behavior.

B. The traumatic event is persistently reexperienced in one (or more) of the following ways:

   1. Recurrent and intrusive distressing recollections of the event, including images, thoughts, or perceptions. **Note:** In young children, repetitive play may occur in which themes or aspects of the trauma are expressed.
   2. Recurrent distressing dreams of the event. **Note:** In children, there may be frightening dreams without recognizable content.
   3. Acting or feeling as if the traumatic event were recurring (includes a sense of reliving the experience, illusions, hallucinations, and dissociative flashback episodes, including those that occur on awakening or when intoxicated). **Note:** In young children, trauma-specific re-enactment may occur.
   4. Intense psychological distress at exposure to internal or external cues that symbolize or resemble an aspect of the traumatic event.
   5. Physiological reactivity on exposure to internal or external cues that symbolize or resemble an aspect of the traumatic event.

C. Persistent avoidance of stimuli associated with the trauma and numbing of general responsiveness (not present before the trauma), as indicated by three (or more) of the following:

   1. Efforts to avoid thoughts, feelings, or conversations associated with the trauma.

2. Efforts to avoid activities, places, or people that arouse recollection of the trauma.
3. Inability to recall an important aspect of the trauma.
4. Markedly diminished interest or participation in significant activities.
5. Feeling of detachment or estrangement from others.
6. Restricted range of affect (e.g., unable to have loving feelings).
7. Sense of a foreshortened future (e.g., does not expect to have a career, marriage, children, or a normal life span).

D. Persistent symptoms of increased arousal (not present before the trauma), as indicated by two (or more) of the following:

1. difficulty falling or staying asleep
2. irritability or outbursts of anger
3. difficulty concentrating
4. hypervigilance
5. exaggerated startle response.

E. Duration of the disturbance (symptoms in Criteria B, C, and D) is more than 1 month.

F. The disturbance causes clinically significant distress or impairment in social, occupational, or other important areas of functioning.

Specify if:

Acute: if duration of symptoms is less than 3 months

Chronic: if duration of symptoms is 3 months or more

Specify if:

With Delayed Onset: if the onset of symptoms is at least 6 months after the stressor

Reprinted with permission from the Diagnostic and Statistical Manual of Mental Disorders, Fourth Edition, Text Revision, Copyright 2000, American Psychiatric Association.

Diminished interest, numbing, and detachment could be considered "negative symptoms".

While traumatic re-experiencing and "negative symptoms" are both traceable to the presence of trauma, it does not mean that they can be approached conceptually in the same manner. An actively distressed and unstable patient is different from the detached and constricted one. We could argue that both states represent regressions in personality functioning, but they are regressions of a different kind. In one instance, we seek to help the patient integrate and modulate their affect and become organized. In the second instance, we are confronting an absence of normal motivation and emotional investment.

The negative symptoms are especially difficult when they have evolved into a chronic phase. The DSM-IV diagnostic scheme does not really deal sufficiently with the chronic phase. It defines the disturbance as chronic if it exceeds three months.

However, in many clinical settings, including those in which pseudoseizures patients are seen, the duration of the traumatic syndromes is measured in years and not months.

Lacking a description of the chronic phase, particularly a chronic phase which spans years or decades, is not a minor problem, because it cannot be assumed that the clinical picture will remain unchanged, either in terms of symptomatology, or the dynamic processes operative in the chronic phase, or with respect to treatment implications.

The recovery of interest and vitality in constricted post-traumatic states which have become chronic is a great challenge. One cannot simply persuade the patient to a livelier stance. This process is not like replacing a lost item. It is much more like re-growing an injured nail, or, in severe cases, rehabilitating an abraded landscape.

Constriction and defensive withdrawal are not high-profile symptoms and are, therefore, more readily overlooked, both as a distinctive diagnostic feature, as well as a focus of treatment. This is unfortunate because, from the standpoint of the patient's quality of life, they are just as disruptive as the high-profile acute symptoms. They represent disengagement from the world. Disengagement is not merely a withdrawal. It represents the undoing of connections which support attachment and achievement.

In addition to not dealing with chronic or partial or complex forms of PTSD, the DSM-IV diagnosis also does not deal sufficiently with one of its important diagnostic features, namely, the impairment in social, occupational or other important areas of functioning (DSM-IV, p. 429). While this feature is listed, there is no elaboration.

Impairment in the social, occupational and other important domains of functioning constitutes a lion's share of traumatic disturbance. It could be argued that the processes which determine social and occupational functioning represent the better part of post-traumatic adaptation. These processes consist of an active interplay between the patient's resources and the traumatic experience. They are the "what" and "how"—i.e. the significant particulars of post-traumatic adaptation.

Given the issues raised in the preceding discussion, how should one approach the description of the post-traumatic stress disorder provided by the DSM-IV so as to derive maximal benefit from it? The symptoms listed in this description are both very numerous and have a very broad range. They include a variety of mood and affective disturbances, a variety of anxiety phenomena, disturbances of arousal, disturbances in the quality of consciousness, sleep problems, a diminished sense of interest, vitality and self-esteem. To this are added problems with concentration and memory. While PTSD is classified as an anxiety disorder, the DSM-IV definition shows a range of disturbance which is far more pervasive and cuts across most major sectors of personality functioning. Given this, it would probably be helpful to think in terms of *post-traumatic transformation of personality* and use various symptoms listed as highlights for possible directions in which this transformation can occur.

In addition to the features described in the preceding discussion, traumatic syndromes presented in this context have a characteristic which we could call "historicity". This feature adds to the complexity of the clinical picture in pseudoseizure patients and is thus to some extent linked to its protean nature.

Historicity of trauma

We shall attempt to illustrate this term by presenting a contrast between two different types of trauma.

The nature of trauma which occurs when a person breaks a leg is very different from trauma stemming from sexual/physical abuse. The former is brief, very explicit, can be localized and externalized readily, there is a clear remedy, and the limits of medical and social responsibility towards the person are clearly defined. Sexual, physical or psychological abuse are not so obvious, and they cannot be readily localized/externalized unless one witnesses the traumatic incidents or there are obvious signs of injury.

In many cases, sexual/physical abuse is not limited to a single event. Even when it is limited, the consequences linger for a time, and defense operations are typically brought forth which can take any number of forms and which also vary from person to person. Thus, trauma stemming from physical/ sexual abuse has a very pronounced component of historicity.

Historicity (as defined in this context) includes not only the traumatic event itself (or, more commonly, a series of events), but also psychological defenses, both conscious and unconscious, which the individual instituted against the impact of trauma. Trauma also changes the baseline of functioning. For example, a traumatized person may respond to a new challenge with diminished vigor and confidence which places him or her at risk to be traumatized again. This is also a component of historicity.

Thus, historicity encompasses a number of different components: the traumatic event, its consequences (both apparent and hidden), as well as the adaptive measures, including unconscious defenses with which the individual protected himself. By this definition, breaking of a leg would be trauma with a low historicity content.

Pseudoseizure patients, by contrast, bring histories which not only contain traumatic events but a good deal of rich history besides. One may encounter distinct traumatic events and their distinct timelines—as well as particular defenses instituted against each trauma. For example, the patient may have suffered multiple instances of childhood abuse, as well as violence sustained during marriage (perhaps multiple marriages). Making sense of this history is somewhat like interpreting the geography of a terrain which contains different topographic features and different layers of soil.

In view of the fact that pseudoseizure patients present with complex histories, which questions can be most profitably asked to reduce the complexity and help us get oriented?

Why does trauma generate specific clinical manifestations which differ so greatly? Why does a particular patient develop one disorder, and not another?

The above questions are very natural and they have a legitimate place in traumatology and the study of pseudoseizures. However, these are not really useful questions in the setting of diagnosis and treatment of post-traumatic pseudoseizures. The first question is not useful, because it often carries an implication that, until and unless one answers why such a diversity of manifestations exists, one cannot competently help the patient. This is not true.

The question which asks why one specific disorder in response to trauma and not some other specific disorder is even more difficult to answer. It is likewise not true that, until one answers that question, one cannot deal with an individual patient.

The more useful question, in our view, is how has this particular patient responded to trauma/loss? The focus is on understanding the dynamics of individual adaptation, whether it is similar to or different from other patients'. This focus has remained unchanged for one hundred years and continues to be valid. It is a historic role and responsibility of therapists.

What to do with protean histories?

Crowded histories, which pseudoseizure patients often present with, can be distracting. They become less distracting if three questions are initially asked:

- Is there a history of trauma or loss?
- Is there chronicity in the clinical picture?
- Is the clinical picture protean?

If the answer to all three of these questions is yes, it is likely that one is dealing with a post-traumatic disturbance. This disturbance may or may not be related to pseudoseizures. However, the presence of post-traumatic disturbance, in and of itself, is an indication for psychotherapy and provides a natural focus for treatment. It sets treatment priority regardless of whether this disturbance is related to pseudoseizures or not.

Sometimes, therapists are afraid to simply deal with the traumatic disturbance unless and until it can be proven that this disturbance is responsible for pseudoseizures. This view is erroneous for several reasons. Typically, the relationship to pseudoseizures—the casual relationship—cannot be established until treatment is well under way. The emergence of causal connections occurs only after a good deal of therapeutic work and is a result of it.

In those cases in which the causal connection between the trauma and pseudoseizures cannot be established, the treatment of the traumatic disturbance is still relevant and inherently valuable.

Finally, it should be noted that traumatic disturbance—regardless of how it is manifested—cannot be simply ignored. It is not an inert collection of historic data. On the contrary, it has a way of exerting influence on the patient's functioning whether this is readily apparent or not. It is unlikely that other therapeutic agenda can be successfully pursued if significant traumatic disturbance is ignored.

The possibility of a traumatic disturbance should be given serious consideration even if one cannot immediately elicit a history of trauma, yet the patient presents with chronic disturbance and a protean clinical picture. It is, of course, true that chronicity and complexity do not, in and of themselves, necessarily imply the presence of trauma. Patients can have complicated histories for other reasons. However, in the tertiary care settings in which pseudoseizure patients are most commonly evaluated and treated, it is a very useful hypothesis.

A lack of coherence in the clinical picture and the protean nature of symptoms become more manageable and less confusing if one uses them as clues to trauma and not as barriers to understanding.

How to conceptualize the nature of trauma?

- Loss
- Regression
- It entails a developmental crisis

In what way is it like a loss?

At the most obvious level, a loss occurs through death or separation from loved ones. Physical, sexual, or psychological abuse also entail a loss, because it is a loss of a relationship (with parent or spouse) which would otherwise be there and which the person needs to function. Trauma can also occur through a loss of stability and security. Disruption of a secure base through abuse and, especially, through war, is a loss, in fact, it can be conceptualized as a whole series of losses.

In what way does trauma entail regression?

Regression is a decrease in the adequacy of functioning which has a reduction in the quality of life as a final outcome. Regression can be mild and transient, or severe and pervasive. Regression can take many forms. A loss of motivation and hope is a form of regression. Overt symptoms, for example, anxiety, depressiveness, and sexual difficulties, are common forms of regression. Symptoms are a signal of regression, because their presence suggests that the person is struggling with some difficulty which he or she has not yet overcome. By this definition, pseudoseizures can be seen as a manifestation of regression, because they cause discomfort and affect the quality of life considerably.

Also, they represent an unconscious and therefore automatic, as opposed to a reasoned strategy of dealing with the traumatic experience. In addition, they are a partial and not a complete solution. They are partly a symptom and partly a solution.

It should be noted, in this context, that not all types of reactions to trauma entail regression. As we have observed earlier, some individuals respond rapidly and effectively, and after they have been challenged, they regroup and move on.

Still others go beyond mere effectiveness. They not only do not allow the traumatic experience to stall their life – they use it creatively so that the traumatic event is no longer an obstacle, but a focal point around which greater understanding of the human condition can arise, in their own life, as well as the life of others. Such a path of post-traumatic adaptation is found in artists, authors, leaders, and individuals who have a charismatic, therapeutic or mentoring function in the lives of others. In this setting, regression is either minimal or it is transient and is followed by creative adaptive processes which enable the person to become more powerful and more effective.

In clinical settings, however, we are often faced with cases of post-traumatic adaptation which do not follow the above course. In addition to the already mentioned examples of regression—namely various symptoms, including pseudoseizure episodes—there are other instances of regression in the setting of pseudoseizure syndromes which are noteworthy. They will be reviewed in the following sections.

Compulsive emotional remembering

Compulsive emotional remembering which is so common in complicated mourning is an instance of regression. It represents a repeated intrusion of poignant affect into the normal baseline of a person' s functioning. This intrusion has a capacity to preempt all other contents of daily life and reduce the person's investment into various life domains with which he or she is and should remain naturally involved. Although compulsive emotional remembering is an important part of the resolution of traumatic experience (or traumatic loss), nevertheless, while it lasts, it can significantly constrict motivation which sustains productive goals.

The intrusive affect and memories tend to follow a somewhat autonomous course. Their expression is difficult to inhibit or direct, both for the person who is experiencing them and for those trying to help them. The regressive quality of compulsive emotional remembering is thus evident both in the intrusive and semi-autonomous nature of affective remembrance, as well as in the inhibition of motivation which supports productive goals.

Borderline syndromes

Clinical picture of individuals who have developed features of borderline syndromes in response to trauma entails multiple instances of regression. Regressions can be viewed as qualitative changes in the manner of relatedness and in the processing of affect.

Affective experience becomes more intense, yet more diffuse and less responsive to ideas and words. It assumes the quality of a drive without a goal.

The nature of relatedness also changes such that the other person is needed urgently as someone who must provide the emotional function of a barrier against the destructive impact of the outside world which is experienced as impinging. The other person functions as a defensive shield against the experience of internal assault, as well as the perceived destructiveness of the outside world. For the regressed patient, the two experiences cannot be separated.

The need to regulate one's affect (and especially, to detoxify intensely negative affective states) through other people is characteristic of a historically earlier level of personality/ affective organization. Although other people remain, to some extent, in the role of a shield throughout our lifetime, the repeated and pervasive regressions to that level of relatedness are characteristic of borderline syndromes.

The need to experience the other person as a filter or a shield against disturbing affective experience is not necessarily obvious. Patients who develop psychotic ideation, delusions or hallucinations, as well as patients who are demented, are readily recognized as having regressed. Traumatic regressions in the level of relatedness, on the other hand, are not clearly recognizable at the outset, and they can occur very abruptly and unexpectedly. They are mostly inferred from the patient's readiness to act out, or to become rapidly disorganized and unable to perform in areas which normally present no difficulty. The patient may present as someone who is simultaneously needy, angry, and confused. A borderline individual comes across as someone who is, paradoxically, both needy and unrelated.

Helping a patient in the regressed state amounts to creating a pontoon bridge or a scaffolding around a house which has temporarily collapsed or is threatening to collapse. Therapeutic intervention—the aim of which is to provide the scaffolding in order to buttress a vulnerable structure—is not very different from the parental involvement with a child who is traversing a developmental stage in which he or she needs to learn to filter his own negative affects and establish his own homeostatic mechanisms. The regression thus presents a challenge which in some ways resembles the challenge of a normative developmental crisis.

The characteristics of a developmental crisis can be summarized as follows. The skill to be acquired is needed for the normal functioning of the personality. The process of learning it cannot be avoided or bypassed without cost to the person. Second, the process of acquiring the function is not automatic—it takes time and cannot be spearheaded. Finally, in order to successfully complete a given developmental stage, input and involvement from others are required.

Borderline regression can thus be viewed, to some extent, as a compressed developmental crisis. In an analogous way, the therapist's response to the patient, involves, to some extent, compressed and symbolic parenting.

Narcissistic injury

Narcissistic injury is a loss of self-coherence in which the sense of self-esteem is abruptly injured. This experience is marked by a poignant sense of loss of value. One has ceased to be valuable in a very unexpected way. A sense of shame is readily evoked in this situation, as well as anger which may be expressed in diverse ways, and which functions to protect the individual from shame. The experience of narcissistic injury may be very brief, or prolonged and chronic.

Narcissistic injury is not limited to a specific type of traumatic experience. For example, it can occur in pseudoseizure patients who were victims of abuse or sexual assault. In our preceding discussions, however, we focused on its role in the dynamics of postconcussive/post-traumatic syndromes, because it has particular significance in that context. Namely, an unacknowledged or unresolved narcissistic injury in that setting may be one of the chief barriers to the patient's getting better. It stalls the patient's life.

Chief features of narcissistic injury—anger and immobilization—can be viewed as forms of regression.

Narcissistic injury is a loss of sense of self as we value it—it is a loss of sense of value of what is unalienably ours. This loss is a regression of a particular kind. It is a sudden loss of a foundation .The individual has the feeling of being robbed, of having the rug pulled from under them. The *experience of self as valuable is a critical source of motivation*—a permanent sponsor of our goals. If this foundation is even transiently withdrawn, immobilization can ensue. Thus, narcissistic injury is frequently accompanied by immobilization.

The anger induced by a sense of shame also has regressive qualities. While normal adults are certainly capable of both anger and shame, the anger induced by shame in response to a narcissistic injury is somewhat different in that the individual is very difficult to soothe and reach through words. It is an anger which is not readily symbolizable.

Narcissistic injury may be brief, yet, while it lasts, its affects seem frozen. There is something very rigid and almost autonomous about the quality of that experience. After the person has recovered and regained a greater sense of coherence, he or she may show a much greater affective range. The shame and anger may be greatly attenuated and replaced by other affects which are more modulated and integrated with other facts of the situation. The prevailing affective climate during the period of narcissistic injury, however, may be as different from the person's normal state as a different geological stratum. This difference makes it a regressive experience.

We defined narcissistic injury as being somewhat like a fault in the foundation of self-experience, a *breach* in the experience of well-being. This situation is similar to a developmental crisis, because the sense of well-being and coherence which was traumatically lost must be recovered, just as during a particular period of self development it must be originally established.

Some forms of narcissistic injury are brief and they can be substantially reversed by a single successful intervention. Thus, the recovery is not necessarily prolonged and elaborate. However, we also often encounter cases in which the narcissistic vulnerability is more pronounced and more entrenched. The recovery in those cases is one of the most significant therapeutic challenges. It essentially requires that substantial portions of the fundamental motivational structure of the personality be somehow rebuilt. The process of rehabilitation recapitulates , albeit in a symbolic and compressed form, the key aspects of the normative development of the self. This implies that the process of rehabilitation requires time and narcissistic supplies need to be available to the individual.

Clinical implications

Why conceptualize trauma, or, more specifically, traumatic disturbance, in terms of the three key components: loss, regression and a developmental crisis?

Trauma, as we characterized it here, is not just the traumatic event, but rather what the patient feels and does as a result of it, and what happens to him or her as a result of it. It is much more of a process than an event.

This process can be conceptualized in different ways. The particular model presented here has several advantages. It is a model which streamlines the task of reviewing the often complex histories of pseudoseizure patients. It imposes organization.

This model reflects our understanding that a loss or active trauma are very common in histories of pseudoseizure patients. Furthermore, it makes explicit the presence of regression.

A search for regression in the clinical history is a very active analytic process which introduces structure. Some regressions are very apparent and some are subtle. In either case, being able to identify regression suggests that at least a rudimentary understanding of the case has been achieved.

The nature of regression determines, to an important extent, the nature of psychopathology. For example, it matters whether a regression is a form of complicated mourning or borderline regression. In the former case, we expect compulsive emotional remembering and a withdrawal from pleasurable activities. While undoubtedly disruptive, these symptoms have different and also less severe implications for the patient's life than regressions which resemble borderline syndromes. The latter involve a loss of capacity to regulate affect, an increased potential for acting out, possible brief psychotic experiences and possible suicidality.

As we observed earlier, not all regressions which occur in the setting of post-traumatic adaptation need to be complex or severe. However, the present model encourages the clinician to approach the history with an expectation that some form of regression might be there.

Understanding the nature of regression is linked to an understanding of defenses which the patient has relied on in order to protect himself or herself against the impact of trauma.

In this model, the concept of regression is intimately tied to the concept of a developmental crisis.

The idea of a developmental crisis is advantageous, because it helps us to deal with the fact that many traumatized individuals who seek help in tertiary care settings—among them pseudoseizure patients—do not (insofar as we are aware) simply get well automatically. This is not to understate the importance of natural processes of psychological healing which do occur whether we are able to understand them or not. We rely on these processes implicitly in any treatment. However, they may not be enough.

The idea of a developmental crisis is meant to help the clinician avoid a common error. This error consists of an expectation that the patient will recover from the traumatic experience more or less automatically, and if he or she does not, there is something fundamentally wrong with them. A corollary to this idea is a notion that normal people recover from whatever trauma happens to befall them, as a matter of course, and that the development of symptomatology is a sign of their pre-existing psychological vulnerability.

While there may be an element of truth in each of these statements, they are not a useful guide in formulating a therapeutic approach to pseudoseizure patients. They are dogmatic statements insofar as they block rather than encourage efforts to understand all we can about the patient's particular response and adaptation. Any particular patient may indeed recover from trauma in a semi-automatic way, after a transient disruption. However, our primary responsibility when faced with a traumatized pseudoseizure patient is not to expect, especially not a priori, such an outcome. Our primary responsibility is to understand the particulars of the patient's case and treat what is most relevant to his or her well-being.

The idea of a developmental crisis also directs us to inquire about particular skills or developmental milestones which the patient needs to re-establish in order to get better. While the person is re-capturing or relearning the traumatically lost developmental milestone, his or her levels of performance will be expected to fluctuate as with any other new task.

From the point of view of the therapist, it is easier to accept the frustrations and the inevitable fluctuations in the patient's recovery if we can conceptualize them as a reactivation of an earlier developmental passage, i.e. as a process which in some way has to do with new learning. Consistent with this view, it is helpful to remember that the process of rehabilitation has the character and the timeline of organic growth.

Summary

Is there a traumatic disturbance?

Taken together, the presence of trauma/or loss, as well a chronicity and complexity of the patient's history, make it likely that one is dealing with a traumatic disturbance. Traumatic disturbance refers specifically to adverse consequences of trauma on the patient's life. It should be noted that the mere presence of trauma in the patient's history does not necessarily indicate a disturbance since a given individual may well have dealt with that event successfully. Nonetheless, in settings in which pseudoseizure cases are evaluated, histories of traumatic disturbance, and not just traumatic events, are sufficiently likely to be relevant. In sum, traumatic disturbance is more likely to be underdiagnosed than to be overdiagnosed.

Characterizing the nature of trauma

Having determined that one is probably dealing with a traumatic disturbance and not merely a history of traumatic events, we can proceed to characterize the nature of trauma. This process includes identifying specific traumatic events and their background.

Next, it is important to identify regressions in functioning. These regressions can be manifested either in active symptoms, or in withdrawal and immobilization, or some combination of both. The presence of regression is often manifested in a protean symptoms picture in which a great deal is happening. One is left with the impression that perhaps too much is happening.

On the other hand, trauma can also lead to a very constricted, or impoverished clinical picture. When faced with such a picture one frequently feels that too little is happening, and that the patient ought to be much more involved, and much more invested. "Too little" in the symptom picture can be the result of defensive constriction and withdrawal which are also forms of regression and their implications are just as serious.

Finally, we are confronting a question as to which issues or milestones in object-relations development, i.e. in the development of affect and relatedness, are most relevant in the particular patient's clinical picture.

Characterizing clinical picture and psychodynamics

- most like complicated mourning?
- most like narcissistic injury?
- most like regression resembling borderline syndromes?

The nature of recovery

Recovery from trauma is frequently referred to as *resolution*. This is a good description since resolution is a process whereby greater clarity is achieved. With increased resolution, the contents of a picture becomes clearer to the observer and objects are more sharply defined.

Greater clarity or articulation of the cause/effect relationship, while very important, is only one aspect of recovery. In treating individuals who have been traumatized we are also often faced with the necessity of re-building in some way that which was traumatically lost. This is a task of a different order. Here, we are concerned not so much with resolution as with restitution.

Restitution is a process of restoring or making good on damage. It entails recreating not just the appearance, but the *substance* of something which was damaged. It is not a palliative process. Rather, it has to do with re-emergence of strength and wholeness. For this to occur, a transformation of some kind is necessary.

How this process operates is not fully understood. From the standpoint of the therapeutic process, we know that an empathic understanding and clarity facilitate restitution. A therapeutic environment could probably be described as one which facilitates restitution.

Recovery as restitution is probably most evident in helping patients who are narcissistically injured. Some forms of narcissistic injury are such that they could be rapidly reversed with a right kind of statement. Such a statement is not an interpretation (although an interpretation can also have a powerfully restitutive character). It is not an attempt at greater clarity, but at restoring wholeness. From the patient's point of view, such an intervention serves to restore access to his own resources of motivation, pleasure and initiative.

Patients experiencing borderline regression are especially threatened with a sense of fragmentation which is complicated by what we referred to earlier as an affective silence. Affective silence entails a sense that one is unable to match oneself to the world, a troubling sense that *one's affects no longer have currency in the world*. Therapeutic intervention in that setting has clearly the character of restitution, of re-establishing a transiently lost foundation.

Words are often thought of as symbols and one of the goals of therapy is to make the patient more capable of symbolizing his affects and experience, instead of erasing them through repression or diverting them into symptoms. Words do function symbolically and the capacity to respond to words as symbols remains crucial to interpersonal adjustment. In borderline regressions and narcissistic injury, however, therapeutic words function more as signals than as symbols. More specifically, they are experienced as *signals of restitution*. A signal is something of immediate relevance and it is affectively more direct. It has a capacity to restore a breach in the experience of the self.

The character of restitution in borderline patients in many ways resembles restoring a weight-bearing wall or a structure so that it is again viable.

The need for restitution in perhaps most easily recognizable in mourning where the manifestations of regression—the loss of confidence and initiative—are obviously linked to a loss. How this process of regression is reversed is not clear. We have at least some degree of confidence that restitution will eventually occur. However, when it does occur, we cannot claim that it has occurred in a straightforward way, the way an empty jug is refilled with water. While recovery appears outwardly as a quantitative change—the patient is less depressed and less immobilized or is more confident and more engaged—it is more likely that a whole series of qualitative changes have taken place. These changes have most probably recreated a network, a new weight-bearing structure perhaps, and not just a single pathway.

Freud discovered that the process of mourning which was not straightforward to begin with might, in some cases, be complicated by the added complexity of the identification with the lost love object, thus setting up a potential for an ongoing conflict. In an effort to adapt to grief, the lost person is retained, not as a passive image or a memory, but as a psychological fact. He or she is retained in a disruptive way, as someone who is, oddly, both an adversary and also a part of oneself. This means that he or she cannot be dealt with simply by passive forgetting, as desirable as this might be.

From the struggles of his patients, Freud gained an empathic access to *the aggressive mantle of grief*—a special hardship of the bereaved. From the unexpected affects of grief he was able to make further intuitive dynamic links to the nature of attachment, specifically an empathic appreciation for the ambivalence felt towards those to whom we are most strongly attached.

In the setting of complicated grief, restitution entails a great deal more than a peaceful attrition of memories and connections with the lost loved person. It amounts to being able to face the fact that affects of grief are essentially *affects of battle.*

It is true that there are cases in which restitution occurs in a simple and reassuring way which outwardly resembles the process of replenishing an empty jug with water. However, from the psychodynamic point of view, i.e. from the standpoint of the patient's experience, adaptation to trauma and loss are really forms of soldiering.

Understanding recovery as restitution is many things. It encompasses an appreciation for the degree to which overcoming the impact of traumatic events is a struggle of a particular kind. It also confers an understanding that restitution represents growth of a special kind and, like other kinds of growth in nature, it has its own intrinsic parameters and its own timelines.

Rehabilitation of trauma could be compared to a rehabilitation of burnt or abraded landscape or a disrupted ecosystem. Different things matter in an ecosystem and they may all follow their own distinct recovery timelines and may require different kinds of resources for recovery. For example, rehabilitating soil is a different kind of process from the one which brings forth the return of birds and other animal life to the recovering site.

Bibliography

American Psychiatric Association, 1994, *Diagnostic and Statistical Manual of Mental Disorders*, 4th edition, Washington, D. C., American Psychiatric Association.

Bergen, D., Daugherty, S. and Eckenfels, E., 1992, Reduction of sexual activities in females taking antiepileptic drugs, *Psychopathology*, 25, 1–4.

Betts, T. and Boden, S., 1992, Diagnosis, management and prognosis of a group of 128 patients with non-epileptic attack disorder: II Previous childhood sexual abuse in the etiology of these disorders, *Seizure*, 1, 27–32.

Bion, Wilfred, R., 1977, *Seven Servants—Four Works by Wilfred R. Bion*, Jason Aronson, Inc., New York, NY.

Bowman, Elizabeth, S., 1993, Etiology and Clinical Course of Pseudoseizures: Relationship to Trauma, Depression and Dissociation, *Psychosomatics*, 34 (4), pp. 333–42.

Breslau, Naomi et al., 1997, Psychiatric Sequelae of Post-Traumatic Stress Disorder in Women, *Archives of General Psychiatry*, 54 (January), pp. 81–7.

Browne, A. and Finkelhor, D., 1986, Impact of child sexual abuse: A review of the research, *Psychological Bulletin*, 99 (1), pp. 66–77.

Carscadon, Mary, A., and Rechtschaffen, Allan, 2000, Monitoring and Staging Human Sleep, in Meir H. Kryger, Thomas Roth, and William C. Dement (eds), *Principles and Practice of Sleep Medicine*, 3rd edition, W. B. Saunders Company—A Harcourt Health Sciences Company, Philadelphia, London and New York, NY, p. 1197.

Cartmill, A. and Betts, T., 1992, Seizure behavior in a patient with post-traumatic stress disorder following rape. Notes on the etiology of pseudoseizures, *Seizure*, 1, pp. 33–6.

Charcot, J. M., 1879, Hystero-epilepsy, in G. Sigerson (trans.), *Lectures on the Diseases of the Nervous System*, Lea, Philadelphia, pp. 247–60.

Davies, M. J. and Frawley, M. G., 1991, Dissociative processes and transference-countertransference paradigms in the psychoanalytically-oriented treatment of adult survivors of childhood sexual abuse, *Psychoanalytic Dialogues*, 2 (1), pp. 5–36.

Ferenczi, Sandor, 1927, *Further Contributions to the Theory and Technique of Psycho-Analysis* (compiled by John Rickman), authorized translation from the German by Jane Isabel Stuttie et al., Boni and Liveright, New York.

Ferenczi, Sandor, 1949, Confusion of Tongues Between the Adult and the Child, *International Journal of Psycho-Analysis*, 30, pp. 225–30.

Festinger, L., 1957, *A Theory of Cognitive Dissonance*, Row and Peterson, Evanston, Illinois.

Freud, Sigmund, 1917, Mourning and Melancholia, in *Sigmund Freud Collected Papers*, Vol. 4, pp. 152–70, authorized translation under the supervision of Joan Riviere, the International Psycho-Analytical Library No.10, edited by Ernest Jones, MD, Basic Books, Inc., New York, NY, 1959.

Freud, Sigmund, 1928, Dostoevsky and Parricide, in *Sigmund Freud Collected Papers*, Vol. 5, pp. 222–42, edited by James Strachey, The International Psycho-Analytical Library, No. 37, edited by Ernest Jones, MD Basic Books, Inc., New York, 1959.

Gabbard, G. O., 1991, commentary on "Dissociative processes and transference-countertransference paradigms" by Davies, M. and Frawley, M. G., *Psychoanalytic Dialogues*, 2 (1), pp. 37–47.

Gabbard, G. O., 1986, The Treatment of the "Special" Patient in a Psychoanalytic Hospital, *International Review of Psychoanalysis*, 13, pp. 333–47.

Garden, F. H., Bontke, C. F. and Hoffman, M., 1990, Sexual functioning and marital adjustment after traumatic brain injury, *Journal of Head Trauma Rehabilitation*, 5 (2), pp. 52–5.

Giovacchini, Peter L., 1976, original reference to "smoothly balanced relationship" in Symbiosis and Intimacy (p. 420), in *International Journal of Psychoanalytic Psychotherapy,* Vol. 5, 1976, edited by Robert Langs and the Editorial Board, Jason Aronson, New York, NY, p. 413–36.

Giovacchini, Peter L., 1976, p. 359, cited by Michael Sperling in Fusional Relations in the Borderline and Normative Realm: Desperate Love (pp. 358–66), in Reuben Fine (ed.), 1989, *Current and Historical Perspectives on the Borderline Patient,* Current Issues in Psychoanalytic Practice—Monographs of the Society for Psychoanalytic Training Number 1, Brunner and Mazel, New York, NY.

Gross, M., 1982, Incest and hysterical seizures, *Medical Hypnoanalysis*, 3, 146–52.

Gutmann, D., 1987, *Reclaimed Powers: Toward a New Psychology of Men and Women in Later Life*, Basic Books, New York, NY.

Horowitz, M., 1986, Stress response syndromes: A review of post-traumatic and adjustment disorders, *Hospital and Community Psychiatry*, 37 (3), pp. 241–9.

Janet, Pierre, 1965, *The Major Symptoms of Hysteria*, Fifteen Lectures Given in the Medical School of Harvard University; 2nd edition with New Matter (Facsimile of 1929 edition), Hafner Publishing Company, New York, NY, and London, 1965.

Jefferson, Thomas, 1826, letter to the mayor of Washington, June 24, in David McCullough, 2001, *John Adams*, Simon and Schuster, London and New York, NY, p. 645.

Jehu, D., 1991, Post-traumatic stress reactions among adults molested as children, *Sexual and Marital Therapy*, 6 (3), pp. 227–43.

Kalogjera, Ikar, et al., 1998, The Narcissistic Couple, in Jon Carlson and Len Sperry (eds), *The Disordered Couple*, Brunner/Mazel Publishers, New York, NY, pp. 207–38.

Kalogjera-Sackellares, D., 1996, Psychological Disturbances in Patients with Pseudoseizures, in Sackellares, J. C. and Berent, S. (eds), *Psychological Disturbances in Epilepsy*, pp. 191–217, Butterworth-Heinemann, Boston, Oxford.

Kalogjera-Sackellares, D. and Sackellares, J. C., 1997a, Personality profiles of patients with pseudoseizures, *Seizure* 6, pp. 1–7.

Kalogjera-Sackellares, D., and Sackellares, J. C., 1997b, Analysis of MMPI patterns in patients with psychogenic pseudoseizures, *Seizure*, 6, pp. 419–27.

Kardiner, A., 1959, Traumatic neuroses of war, in Silvano Arieti (ed), *American Handbook of Psychiatry*, 1, Basic Books, New York, pp. 245–57.

Kay, Jerald, 1990, Traumatic Deidealization and the Future of Medicine, *Journal of the American Medical Association*, Vol. 263 (4), pp. 572–3.

Kernberg, Otto F., 1976, *Object Relations Theory and Clinical Psychoanalysis*, Jason Aronson, Inc., New York, NY.

Kessler, Ronald C., et al., 1995, Post-Traumatic Stress Disorder in the National Comorbidity Survey, *Archives of General Psychiatry*, 52 (December), pp. 1048–60.

Kohut, Heinz, 1972, Thoughts on Narcissism and Narcissistic Rage, *The Psychoanalytic Study of the Child*, Vol. 27, pp. 360–400.

Kohut, Heinz, 1984, *How Does Analysis Cure?*, (edited by Arnold Goldberg with the collaboration of Paul Stepansky), University of Chicago Press, Chicago, Illinois and London, p. 194.

Kohut, Heinz, 1987, *The Kohut Seminars on Self Psychology and Psychotherapy with Adolescents and Young Adults* (edited by Miriam Elson), W. W. Norton & Company, London and New York, NY.

Kohut, Heinz, 1996, *Heinz Kohut—The Chicago Institute Lectures* (edited by Paul Tolpin and Marian Tolpin), Analytic Press, Hillsdale, NJ, p. 289.

Kohut, Heinz and Wolf, Ernst S., 1978, The Disorders of the Self and Their Treatment: An Outline, *International Journal of Psycho-Analysis and Bulletin of the International Psycho-Analytical Association*, Vol. 59, pp. 413–25.

Kosteljanetz, M. et al., 1981, Sexual and hypothalamic dysfunction in the postconcussional syndrome, *Acta Neurologica Scandinavica*, 63, pp. 169–80.

Krystal, H., 1970, Trauma and the stimulus barrier, paper presented at the annual meeting of the Psychoanalytic Association, San Francisco (quoted in Krystal, 1981).

Krystal, H., 1981, The aging survivor of the Holocaust, Integration and self-healing in post-traumatic states, *Journal of Geriatric Psychiatry*, 14 (2), pp. 165–89.

Levinson, D. J., 1977, The mid-life transition: A period in adult psychosocial development, *Psychiatry*, 40, pp. 99–112.

Mahler, Margaret, 1968, On Human Symbiosis and the Vicissitudes of Individuation, Vol. 1, Infantile Psychosis International Psycho-Analytical Library, No 82, International Universities Press, Inc., New York, NY.

Mahler, Margaret, 1972, Rapprochement subphase of the separation-individuation process, *The Psychoanalytic Quarterly*, Vol. 41 (4), pp. 487–506.

Masterson, James F., 1987, Borderline and Narcissistic Disorders: An Integrated Developmental Object Relations Approach, in James Grotstein, Marion F. Solomo, and Joan A. Lang (eds), *The Borderline Patient: Emerging Concepts in Diagnosis, Psychodynamics and Treatment*, Vol. 1, Analytic Press, London and Hillsdale, NJ.

McDade, G. and Brown, S. W., 1992, Non-epileptic seizures: Management and predictive factors of outcome, *Seizure*, 1, pp. 7–10.

Nemiah, J. C., 1973, Psychology and psychosomatic illness: Reflections on theory and research methodology, *Psychotherapy and Psychosomatics*, 22, pp. 106–11.

Ornstein, Paul, H. and Ornstein, Anna, 1977, On the Continuing Evolution of Psychoanalytic Psychotherapy: Reflections and Predictions, *The Annual of Psychoanalysis*, 5, pp. 329–70, a publication of the Chicago Institute for Psychoanalysis, International Universities Press, New York, NY.

Poe, Edgar Allan, 2002a, The Song (reference to "kindling light"), in *The Complete Tales and Poems of Edgar Allan Poe*, Castle Books, Edison, NJ.

Poe, Edgar Allan, 2002b, (reference to "resembling nothing that is ours") in The City in the Sea, in *The Complete Tales and Poems of Edgar Allan Poe*, Castle Books, Edison, NJ.

Prigatano, G. P., 1992, Personality disturbances associated with traumatic brain injury, *Journal of Consulting and Clinical Psychology*, Vol. 60 (3), pp. 360–8.

Pritchard, P. B., 1980, Hyposexuality: A complication of complex partial epilepsy, *Transactions of the American Neurological Association*, 105, pp. 193–5.

Reik, Theodor, 1940, *From Thirty Years with Freud* (trans. Richard Winston), Greenwood Press, Westport, CT, p. 10 of Preface.

Rinsley, Donald B., 1977, An Object-Relations View of Borderline Personality, in Peter Hartcollis (ed.), *Borderline Personality Disorders: The Concept, The Syndrome, The Patient*, International Universities Press, Inc., New York, NY, pp. 47–70.

Rousseau, Jean-Jacques, 1913, *The Social Contract and Discourses* (translated with an Introduction by. G. D. H. Cole), E. P. Dutton & Company, Inc., New York, NY, and J. M. Dent and Sons Ltd, London.

Schlenger, W. E., et al., 1992, The Prevalence of post-traumatic stress disorder in the Vietnam generation: A multimethod, multisource assessment of psychiatric disorder, *Journal of Traumatic Stress*, 5 (3), pp. 333–63.

Shapiro, J. P., 1991, Interviewing children about psychological issues associated with sexual abuse, *Psychotherapy*, Spring 28, pp. 55–66.

Sifneos, P. E., Afpfel-Savitz, R. and Frankel, F. H., 1977, The phenomenon of alexithymia: Observations in neurotic and psychosomatic patients, *Psychotherapy and Psychosomatics*, 28, pp. 47–57.

Stern, Donnel B., 1977, *Unformulated Experience: From Dissociation to Imagination in Psychoanalysis*, Analytic Press, Hillsdale, NJ.

Strozier, Charles B., 2001, *Heinz Kohut—The Making of a Psychoanalyst*, Farrar, Straus, and Giroux, New York, NY, pp. 330–1.

Swenson, Charles R., 1986, Forms of Fusion, (p. 367–76), in Reuben Fine (ed.), *Current and Historical Perspectives on the Borderline Patient*, Current Issues in Psychoanalytic Practice —Monographs of the Society for Psychoanalytic Training, 1989, No.1, Brunner/Mazel Publishers, New York, NY.

Taylor, D. C., 1969, Sexual behavior and temporal lobe epilepsy, *Archives of Neurology*, 21, pp. 510–16.

Van Der Kolk, B. A. and Ducey, C. P., 1989, The psychological processing of traumatic experience: Rorschach patterns in PTSD, *Journal of Traumatic Stress*, 2 (3), pp. 259–74.

Winnicott, D. W., 1965, *The Maturational Processes and the Facilitating Environment: Studies in the Theory of Emotional Development*, International Universities Press, New York, NY.

Index

USA & Canada *orders to:*
Crown House Publishing
P.O. Box 2223, Williston, VT 05495-2223, USA
Tel: 877-925-1213, Fax: 802-864-7626
E-mail: info@CHPUS.com
www.CHPUS.com

UK & Rest of World *orders to:*
The Anglo American Book Company Ltd
Crown Buildings, Bancyfelin, Carmarthen, Wales SA33 5ND
Tel: +44 (0)1267 211880/211886, Fax: +44 (0)1267 211882
E-mail: books@anglo-american.co.uk
www.anglo-american.co.uk

Australasia *orders to:*
Footprint Books Pty Ltd
Unit 4/92A Mona Vale Road, Mona Vale NSW 2103, Australia
Tel: +61 (0) 2 9997 3973, Fax: +61 (0) 2 9997 3185
E-mail: info@footprint.com.au
www.footprint.com.au

Singapore *orders to:*
Publishers Marketing Services Pte Ltd
10-C Jalan Ampas #07-01
Ho Seng Lee Flatted Warehouse, Singapore 329513
Tel: +65 6256 5166, Fax: +65 6253 0008
E-mail: info@pms.com.sg
www.pms.com.sg

Malaysia *orders to:*
Publishers Marketing Services Pte Ltd
Unit 509, Block E, Phileo Damansara 1, Jalan 16/11
46350 Petaling Jaya, Selangor, Malaysia
Tel : 03 7955 3588, Fax : 03 7955 3017
E-mail: pmsmal@po.jaring.my
www.pms.com.sg

South Africa *orders to:*
Everybody's Books
Box 201321 Durban North 401, 1 Highdale Road,
25 Glen Park, Glen Anil 4051, KwaZulu NATAL, South Africa
Tel: +27 (0) 31 569 2229, Fax: +27 (0) 31 569 2234
E-mail: ebbooks@iafrica.com